AF614684

Loss of Vision

Edited by Mateja Jagić and Ratimir Lazić

Published in London, United Kingdom

Loss of Vision
http://dx.doi.org/10.5772/intechopen.104342
Edited by Mateja Jagić and Ratimir Lazić

Contributors
Aji Kunnath Devadas, Andreas Fricke, Ante Barišić, Anujeet Paul, Ao Miao, Dino Šabanović, Jie Xu, Karsten Klabe, Lucija Žerjav, Maja Bohač, Mateja Jagić, Meena Kumari Ramesh, Navaneeth Krishna, Niranjan Karthik Senthil Kumar, Peimin Lin, Prajnya Ray, Prasanna Venkatesh Ramesh, Ramesh Rajasekaran, Sara Blazhevska, Shruthy Vaishali Ramesh, Tianyu Zheng, Yi Lu

First published in London, United Kingdom, 2024 by IntechOpen
IntechOpen is the global imprint of INTECHOPEN LIMITED, registered in England and Wales, registration number: 11086078, 167-169 Great Portland Street, London, W1W 5PF, United Kingdom

British Library Cataloguing-in-Publication Data
A catalogue record for this book is available from the British Library

Additional hard and PDF copies can be obtained from orders@intechopen.com

Loss of Vision
Edited by Mateja Jagić and Ratimir Lazić
p. cm.
Print ISBN 978-1-83768-873-9
Online ISBN 978-1-83768-874-6
eBook (PDF) ISBN 978-1-83768-875-3

For EU product safety concerns:
IN TECH d.o.o., Prolaz Marije Krucifikse Kozulić 3, 51000 Rijeka, Croatia,
info@intechopen.com or visit our website at intechopen.com.

Meet the editors

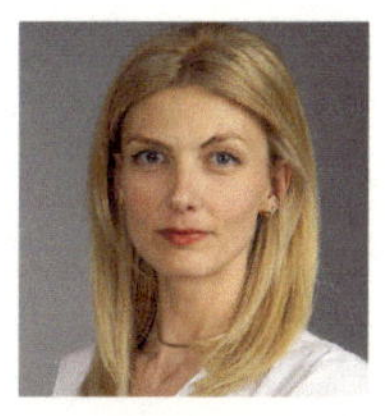

Mateja Jagić graduated from the School of Medicine, University of Osijek, while she completed her ophthalmology and optometry residency training program in 2017 under the mentorship of Professor Iva Dekaris. Since 2011, she works at the Specialty Hospital of Ophthalmology Svjetlost in the Department of Refractive Surgery and the Corneal Department. Training in the field of corneal refractive surgery began under the mentorship of Assistant Professor Maja Bohač, and so far, she has performed several thousand laser surgeries, including PRK, LASIK, and lenticule extraction. Regarding scientific education, she completed her postgraduate study in biomedicine and health at the Faculty of Medicine of the University of Zagreb, and in January 2019 she defended her doctoral dissertation thesis entitled "Visible Outcome after Implantation of Multifocal Intraocular Lenses" in the process of obtaining Ph.D. status. Mateja Jagić is a member of the European Association for Cataract and Refractive Surgery and the Croatian Society for Cataract and Refractive Surgery and regularly participates in annual meetings. She also participates as an educator in corneal refractive surgery at the annual meetings of those associations. She is a co-author of several scientific and professional papers in international journals cited in CC and in the field of refractive surgery. She has participated in several clinical studies for treatment protocols for dry eye disease and novel refractive surgery methods of lenticular extraction.

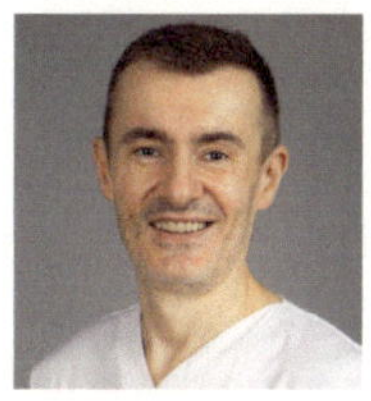

Professor Ratimir Lazić graduated from the School of Medicine University of Zagreb and completed a residency in ophthalmology under the mentorship of Professor Nikica Gabrić. He completed his vitreo-retinal surgery fellowship at the Svjetlost Eye Hospital and holds the position of Retina Department head, where he carries out his professional activity performing procedures such as minimally invasive vitrectomy, combined vitrectomy and cataract surgery, and iris-claw and phakic IOL implantation. In Croatia, he was one of the first to perform bimanual minimally invasive 23 and 25-gauge vitrectomy with chandelier light and using vital dyes (Dual Blue and Brilliant peel) and high-speed cutters. Regarding scientific education, he has completed the postgraduate course in molecular biology at the School of Science, University of Zagreb, where he earned his master's of science degree, and he earned his Ph.D. in the treatment of age-related macular degeneration at the School of Medicine, University of Rijeka, where he holds the position of clinical associate professor. He teaches postgraduate courses in ophthalmology at the Schools of Medicine in Zagreb and Rijeka. So far, he has published 14 papers indexed in CC, with the most important pioneering papers on the treatment of ARMD and DME. For several years he has been acting as an investigator in various multicultural randomized studies in the development of new retinal drugs. He has been a full member of the American Society of Retinal Specialists since 2005 and regularly participates in the annual meetings since 2006.

Contents

Preface

Of the nearly 2.2 billion visually impaired people worldwide, nearly 1 billion face untreated or preventable visual impairment or blindness. Today it is estimated that more than 80% of visual impairment globally can be avoided through prevention, treatment, or cure. Efficient prevention and intervention are vital to mitigate the consequences of visual impairment, where immediate action is crucial for reducing the lasting socioeconomic effects of visual loss. Despite the multifactorial etiology, in this book, we have focused on glaucoma and cataracts as some of the leading causes of visual impairment and blindness globally.

The glaucoma section gives attention to the surgical techniques of canaloplasty and trabeculoplasty, as well as a holistic approach for evaluating and determining glaucomatous damage and its progression. The cataract section focuses on surgical techniques in challenging cases of microphthalmic eyes for achieving satisfactory surgical outcomes. Furthermore, one of the topics we discuss is visual outcomes and patient satisfaction after multifocal IOL implantation, the issue of residual refractive error, and providing surgical options for refractive correction in those patients with corneal laser surgery.

The goal of the book's editors has been to provide clinically relevant overviews as well as future perspectives in the fields of glaucoma, cataract, and refractive surgery. All potential researchers and clinicians who are interested in visual impairment as a global health issue will hopefully find the book interesting. We also hope that readers will find this book useful for the purpose for which it was created with the help and support of the outstanding authors, who invested their time and care in their chapters.

Mateja Jagić
Refractive Surgery and Cornea Department,
University Eye Hospital Svjetlost,
Zagreb, Croatia

Ratimir Lazić
Retina Department,
University Eye Hospital Svjetlost,
Zagreb, Croatia

Section 1

Introduction

Chapter 1

Introductory Chapter: Loss of Vision

Mateja Jagić and Maja Bohač

1. Introduction

Today, it is estimated that nearly one billion people face preventable or untreated visual impairment. The impact of vision loss affects all age groups but particularly the elderly population. Among this cohort, reduced visual acuity has a multi-factorial etiology, including refractive error, cataracts, glaucoma, age-related macular degeneration, and diabetic retinopathy. Statistical projections indicate that the upcoming decades will witness a twofold rise in the number of adults with age-related visual impairments, a trend mostly attributed to the aging global population. Moreover, the surge in chronic diseases like diabetes significantly contributes to an increasing visually impaired population.

In younger individuals, however, congenital cataracts and premature retinopathy stand out as the main culprits of early vision loss. Left undiagnosed, these conditions can result in reduced eyesight or even total blindness, subsequently impacting the psychomotor development and education of the affected children.

Efficient prevention and intervention are vital to mitigate the consequences of visual impairment. Immediate action is crucial to reducing the lasting socioeconomic effects of visual loss, which includes a lower quality of life due to reduced productivity and workforce engagement, to list a few examples.

2. Terminology

Specific terminology has evolved to better define eligibility for disability benefits and rehabilitation training of individuals affected by vision loss. As per the World Health Organization's (WHO) International Classification of Diseases definition (ICD-11), low vision is defined by a visual acuity (VA) of ≤6/18 in the better eye or a visual field (VF) of <10° after medical treatments or with visual aids. Total blindness is indicated by *no light perception* (NLP), affecting around 15% of those with eye disorders. *Legal blindness*, as defined by the United States Social Security Administration (SSA), refers to a best-corrected visual acuity (BCVA) of ≤20/200 or VF of ≤20° in the better eye. Visual impairment, on the other hand, is a term describing decreased visual function, which affects the ability to perform normal activities. Rather than using visual acuity or visual field thresholds, visual impairment is defined focusing only on visual function [1–5].

Based on visual acuity and/or visual field of the better seeing eye, visual impairment has been classified into categories proposed by the WHO and ICD (**Table 1**).

 IntechOpen

Visual impairment grade	Best corrected visual acuity (BCVA)	Visual field range (spatial extent)
Normal	20/10–20/25	
Near normal	20/30–20/60	
Moderate	20/70–20/160	
Severe	20–200 – 20/400	11–20°
Profound	20/500–20/1000	6–10°
Near total	Counting fingers – Light perception	≤ 5°
Total	No light perception	No light perception

Table 1.
Visual impairment classification and grading.

3. Etiology

Visual impairment arises from a diverse set of conditions, involving genetic, congenital, and acquired factors. As highlighted in The WHO World Report of Vision, cataracts, uncorrected refractive errors, age-related macular degeneration, glaucoma, diabetic retinopathy, and trachoma represent the primary contributors to global blindness.

4. Epidemiology

Globally, in accordance with the WHO, over 2.2 billion individuals experience distant or near visual impairment. Among this population, approximately one billion people suffer from visual impairment that could have been prevented or requires therapeutic attention. The primary factors contributing to distance vision impairment or blindness include cataracts (94 million), refractive error (88.4 million), age-related macular degeneration (8 million), glaucoma (7.7 million), and diabetic retinopathy (3.9 million) [6, 7].

In terms of near vision impairment, the predominant issue is presbyopia, impacting a staggering 826 million individuals [8, 9].

The prevalence of blindness is disproportionately higher in developing countries, primarily due to rapid population growth, limited access to ophthalmologic services, cost constraints, and lower education levels. The latter may explain why females are more susceptible to acquiring visual impairments than males [10, 11]. Notably, nearly 90% of blind individuals are indigenous to developing nations.

Moreover, roughly 82% of blind individuals are over the age of 50. Although the adult and senior population is at risk for many debilitating ocular morbidities, childhood blindness is also a significant economic burden, affecting an estimated 1.4 million blind children under 15 years old. Given the projected global population growth to 9.7 billion by 2050, alongside the inevitability of population aging, addressing vision impairment takes first place on the global health agenda [12].

Interestingly, the causes of preventable blindness over the last three decades have changed. The shift has been one away from infectious diseases like trachoma and onchocerciasis toward non-communicable eye diseases (NCED), such as glaucoma, diabetic retinopathy, and age-related macular degeneration (AMD). This shift can be attributed to changing lifestyles and healthcare trends in middle- and low-income nations [7, 8, 13, 14].

5. Presentation and evaluation

Vision loss can manifest gradually or suddenly, leading to a diverse set of possible visual outcomes, including central or peripheral vision loss, overall blurriness, reduced contrast sensitivity, color vision issues, night blindness, glare, or photophobia. The extent of these effects depends on the underlying cause of the vision loss [15].

Obtaining accurate patient history, in addition to a comprehensive clinical assessment, is crucial to successful patient diagnosis and optimal therapy. An effective eye examination should consist of testing for visual acuity, visual field, extraocular muscle movement, pupil sensitivity, binocular vision, intraocular pressure, slit lamp analysis of the anterior segment, and a dilated fundus examination for posterior segment evaluation. However, formal visual field assessment, color vision and contrast sensitivity testing, optical coherence tomography, fluorescein angiography, visual evoked potential, electroretinography, electrooculography, and genetic testing might be additional diagnostic tools essential to accurately diagnose ocular diseases, monitor their progression, and determine patient-appropriate treatment strategies [16].

Those comprehensive eye exams are crucial to prevent, detect, treat, and manage conditions that can cause blindness. These exams should go beyond visual acuity assessments for basic lens prescriptions and include in-depth evaluations of ocular health.

6. Prognosis

The outcome of vision loss depends on the condition at hand, either remaining stable or worsening over time. For instance, age-related macular degeneration mostly affects central vision without leading to total blindness, whereas retinitis pigmentosa begins with peripheral vision loss, progresses to central vision loss, and can eventually result in complete blindness. Timely detection, accurate diagnosis, and appropriate treatment can prevent blindness caused by such conditions. For this reason, it is strongly advised for people of all ages to undergo a comprehensive eye exam every 1–2 years and become proactive in sight-preserving programs that may be offered by their healthcare providers. Also, there are many programs that provide free comprehensive vision and eye health assessments to infants within their first year of life as well as screening and prevention program for children to improve the public health infrastructure supporting the early detection of children's vision problems [17–20].

6.1 Achieving universal coverage for eye health and improving quality of life

Numerous global, national, and local organizations are actively promoting eye health awareness, improving healthcare accessibility, and tackling blindness. Extensive worldwide research programs aim to understand the causes of various eye conditions leading to permanent vision loss and develop effective protocols to better control and treat blinding conditions. The WHO plays a leading role in monitoring such trends, coordinating anti-blindness initiatives [21].

The impact of vision loss on one's quality of life is undeniable. For this reason, vision rehabilitation offers solutions to the functional challenges encountered by individuals with poor vision, including effective use of their residual vision through visual aids and skills training. Moreover, ophthalmologists and optometrists with specialized training in vision rehabilitation have learned to evaluate the patient functional complaints and assess vision thereafter. Such rehabilitation services aim to enhance the quality of life for those with low vision, addressing physical, social, functional, and psychosocial aspects and improving participation in fulfilling basic patient functional needs [22, 23].

Unfortunately, global statistics indicate that only 5–10% of individuals requiring vision rehabilitation services have access to them. Various barriers, including inconsistent service delivery, lack of awareness, mobility issues, language barriers, and inadequate referrals, prevent patient access to better ocular healthcare. Low vision services in developing and developed countries, when compared, reveal distinct challenges [24, 25].

Developing nations face issues like information scarcity, lack of eye health professionals, and uneven service distribution [26], notably in the eastern Mediterranean region, where service availability varies from none to ≤10%. Financial constraints further limit services, often leading the healthcare systems dependent on non-governmental organizations for support [27].

In developed countries, incomplete services result from insufficient data on disease prevalence and causes of blindness and low vision. In high-income region, such as North America and Canada, ophthalmologists serve as the primary referral sources that direct patients to low vision service centers [28]. However, more than just poor vision is usually required to prompt such referrals. Therefore, even in developed countries, inadequate education in vision rehabilitation, high costs associated with misdiagnoses, and a lack of specialized services impact patient vision. A multidisciplinary approach is essential for complete patient assessment but is often not fully implemented. Ultimately, the need for specialized rehabilitation services remains crucial in both developing and developed nations [29].

On another note, data scarcity regarding rehabilitation coverage in developing countries highlights the importance of prioritizing data collection. The Universal Health Coverage study suggested prioritizing data collection in this field [30]. Most studies lack specific clinical diagnoses, and there is therefore a call for comprehensive and accurate data collection [30, 31].

To address the challenges in eye care, such as inequalities in the coverage and quality of prevention, treatment and rehabilitation services, and poor integration of eye-care services into health systems, WHO published *World report on vision* in October 2019 [32]. Endorsing this approach, *The Lancet Global Health Commission on Global Eye Health* [33] proposed ways for advancing health systems toward delivering high-quality integrated eye care within universal health by implementing strategies for the effective integration of eye health services between the primary, secondary, and tertiary levels to improve referral pathways, therefore ensuring recognition of those who need secondary care.

Low-vision rehabilitation services should be available to help patients maximize their residual vision, maintain their independence, and improve their quality of life. These services are provided by a multidisciplinary team of low-vision professionals including optometrists or ophthalmologists, low vision therapists, occupational therapists, orientation and mobility specialists, vocational rehabilitation specialists, rehabilitation teachers, social workers, and other rehabilitation professionals. It is important to recognize that blindness, regardless of the degree, carries significant morbidity and that addressing the challenges of vision loss necessitates a comprehensive interdisciplinary effort to achieve utmost effectiveness in managing and maximizing patient vision and well-being [29–31].

Author details

Mateja Jagić* and Maja Bohač
University Eye Hospital Svjetlost, Zagreb, Croatia

*Address all correspondence to: mateja.jagic@svjetlost.hr

References

[1] Dandona L, Dandona R. Revision of visual impairment definitions in the international statistical classification of diseases. BMC Medicine. 2006;**4**:7. DOI: 10.1186/1741-7015-4-7

[2] Organization WH. Diseases of the eye and adnexa international statistical classification of diseases and related health problems, 10th revision (ICD-10). 2007

[3] Word Health Organization. Global data on visual impairment. 2010. Available from: http:// www.whoint/blindness/ GLOBALDATAFINALforwebpdf

[4] World Health Organization. World Report on Vision. Geneva, Switzerland: WHO; 2019

[5] WHO. World Health Organization fact sheet. Blindness and vision impairment. 2022. [Accessed: April 20, 2023]. Available from: https://www.who.int/news-room/fact-sheets/detail/blindness-and-visual-impairment

[6] Steinmetz JD, Bourne RRA, Briant PS, Flaxman SR, Taylor HR, Jonas JB, et al. Causes of blindness and vision impairment in 2020 and trends over 30 years, and prevalence of avoidable blindness in relation to VISION 2020: The right to sight: An analysis for the global burden of disease study. The Lancet Global Health. 2021;**9**:e144-e160. DOI: 10.1016/S2214-109X(20)30489-7

[7] Keel S, Cieza A. Rising to the challenge: Estimates of the magnitude and causes of vision impairment and blindness. The Lancet Global Health. 2021;**9**(2):e100-e101. DOI: 10.1016/S2214-109X(21)00008-5

[8] GBD 2019 Blindness and Vision Impairment Collaborators, Vision Loss Expert Group of the Global Burden of Disease Study. Causes of blindness and vision impairment in 2020 and trends over 30 years, and prevalence of avoidable blindness in relation to VISION 2020: The right to sight: An analysis for the global burden of disease study. The Lancet Global Health. 2021;**9**(2):e144-e160. DOI: 10.1016/S2214-109X(20)30489-7

[9] Fricke TR, Tahhan N, Resnikoff S, Papas E, Burnett A, Ho SM, et al. Global prevalence of presbyopia and vision impairment from uncorrected presbyopia: Systematic review, meta-analysis, and modelling. Ophthalmology. Oct 2018;**125**(10):1492-1499

[10] Bourne RRA, Flaxman SR, Braithwaite T. Magnitude, temporal trends, and projections of the global prevalence of blindness and distance and near vision impairment: A systematic review and meta-analysis. The Lancet Global Health. 2017;**5**:e888-e897

[11] Abou-Gareeb I, Lewallen S, Bassett K, Courtright P. Gender and blindness: A meta-analysis of population-based prevalence surveys. Ophthalmic Epidemiology. 2001;**8**:39-56

[12] Vollset SE, Goren E, Yuan CW, Cao J, Smith AE, Hsiao T, et al. Fertility, mortality, migration, and population scenarios for 195 countries and territories from 2017 to 2100: A forecasting analysis for the global burden of disease study. Lancet. 2020;**396**(10258):1285-1306. DOI: 10.1016/S0140-6736(20)30677-2. Epub 2020 Jul 14

[13] GBD 2019 Blindness and Vision Impairment Collaborators, Vision Loss

Expert Group of the Global Burden of Disease Study. Trends in prevalence of blindness and distance and near vision impairment over 30 years: An analysis for the global burden of disease study. The Lancet Global Health. 2021;**9**(2):e130-e143. DOI: 10.1016/S2214-109X(20)30425-3. Epub 2020 Dec 1

[14] Yang X, Chen H, Zhang T, Yin X, Man J, He Q, et al. Global, regional, and national burden of blindness and vision loss due to common eye diseases along with its attributable risk factors from 1990 to 2019: A systematic analysis from the global burden of disease study 2019. Aging (Albany NY). 2021;**13**(15):19614-19642. DOI: 10.18632/aging.203374 Epub 2021 Aug 9

[15] Raharja A, Whitefield L. Clinical approach to vision loss: A review for general physicians. Clinical Medicine (London, England). 2022;**22**(2):95-99. DOI: 10.7861/clinmed.2022-0057

[16] Lennie P, Van Hemel SB. The National Research Council (US) committee on disability determination for individuals with visual impairments. In: Visual Impairments: Determining Eligibility for Social Security Benefits. Washington (DC): National Academies Press (US); 2002. Available from: https://www.ncbi. nlm.nih.gov/books/NBK207559/

[17] Fontana C, De Carli A, Ricci D, Dessimone F, Passera S, Pesenti N, et al. Effects of early intervention on visual function in preterm infants: A randomized controlled trial. Frontiers in Pediatrics. 2020;**8**:291. DOI: 10.3389/fped.2020.00291

[18] Nottingham Chaplin PK, Baldonado K, Bergren MD, Lyons SA, Murphy MK, Bradford GE. 12 components of a strong vision health system of care: Part 2-vision screening tools and procedures and vision health for children with special health care needs. NASN School Nurse. 2019;**34**(4):195-201. DOI: 10.1177/1942602X19851724

[19] Nottingham Chaplin PK, Baldonado K, Bergren MD, Lyons SA, Murphy MK, Bradford GE. 12 components of a strong vision health system of care: Part 3-standardized approach for rescreening. NASN School Nurse. 2020;**35**(1):10-14. DOI: 10.1177/1942602X19890470 Epub 2019 Nov 28

[20] Rudnicka AR, Kapetanakis VV, Wathern AK, Logan NS, Gilmartin B, Whincup PH, et al. Global variations and time trends in the prevalence of childhood myopia, a systematic review and quantitative meta-analysis: Implications for aetiology and early prevention. The British Journal of Ophthalmology. 2016;**100**(7):882-890. DOI: 10.1136/bjophthalmol-2015-307724 Epub 2016 Jan 22

[21] World Health Organisation. International Standards for Vision Rehabilitation: Report of the International Consensus Universal Access to Low Vision Rehabilitation. Rome: The International Agency for the Prevention of Blindness; 2015. Available from: www.iapb.org/resources/international-consensus-conference-vision-rehabilitation-standards/

[22] van Nispen RM, Virgili G, Hoeben M, Langelaan M, Klevering J, Keunen JE, et al. Low vision rehabilitation for better quality of life in visually impaired adults. Cochrane Database of Systematic Reviews. 2020;**1**(1):CD006543. DOI: 10.1002/14651858.CD006543.pub2

[23] Agarwal R, Tripathi A. Current modalities for low vision rehabilitation. Cureus. 2021;**13**(7):e16561. DOI: 10.7759/cureus.16561

[24] Sivakumar P, Vedachalam R, Kannusamy V, Odayappan A, Venkatesh R, Dhoble P, et al. Barriers in utilisation of low vision assistive products. Eye (London, England). 2020;**34**(2):344-351. DOI: 10.1038/s41433-019-0545-5. Epub 2019 Aug 6

[25] Chiang PP, O'Connor PM, Le Mesurier RT, Keeffe JE. A global survey of low vision service provision. Ophthalmic Epidemiology. 2011;**18**(3):109-121. DOI: 10.3109/09286586.2011.560745

[26] Forrest SL, Mercado CL, Engmann CM, Stacey AW, Hariharan L, Khan S, et al. Does the current global health agenda lack vision? Global Health, Science and Practice. 2023;**11**(1):e2200091. DOI: 10.9745/GHSP-D-22-00091

[27] GBD 2015 Eastern Mediterranean Region Vision Loss Collaborators. Burden of vision loss in the eastern Mediterranean region, 1990-2015: Findings from the global burden of disease 2015 study. International Journal of Public Health. 2018;**63**(Suppl. 1):199-210. DOI: 10.1007/s00038-017-1000-7. Epub 2017 Aug 3

[28] Gold D, Zuvela B, Hodge WG. Perspectives on low vision service in Canada: A pilot study. Canadian Journal of Ophthalmology. 2006;**41**(3):348-354. DOI: 10.1139/I06-025

[29] Wang BZ, Pesudovs K, Keane MC, Daly A, Chen CS. Evaluating the effectiveness of multidisciplinary low-vision rehabilitation. Optometry and Vision Science. 2012;**89**:1399-1408. DOI: 10.1097/OPX.0b013e3182678d82

[30] GBD 2019 Universal Health Coverage Collaborators. Measuring universal health coverage based on an index of effective coverage of health services in 204 countries and territories, 1990-2019: A systematic analysis for the global burden of disease study 2019. Lancet. 2020;**396**(10258):1250-1284. DOI: 10.1016/S0140-6736(20)30750-9. Epub 2020 Aug 27

[31] Bright T, Wallace S, Kuper H. A systematic review of access to rehabilitation for people with disabilities in low- and middle-income countries. International Journal of Environmental Research and Public Health. 2018;**15**(10):2165. DOI: 10.3390/ijerph15102165

[32] WHO. World report on vision. 2019 [Accessed: May 20, 2023]. Available from: https://www.who.int/publications/i/item/world-report-on-vision

[33] Burton MJ et al. The lancet Global Health Commission on global eye health: Vision beyond 2020. The Lancet Global Health. 2021;**9**(4):e489-e551. DOI: 10.1016/S2214-109X(20)30488-5. Epub 2021 Feb 16

Section 2

Glaucoma

Chapter 2

TIPRA – Three-Dimensional Integrated Progression Analyser: A New World Programme Exploring the Structure-Function Correlation in Glaucoma Using a Holistic 3-Dimensional Approach

Prasanna Venkatesh Ramesh, Anujeet Paul, Shruthy Vaishali Ramesh, Niranjan Karthik Senthil Kumar, Prajnya Ray, Aji Kunnath Devadas, Navaneeth Krishna, Meena Kumari Ramesh and Ramesh Rajasekaran

Abstract

Glaucoma is a chronic, progressive eye disease that causes irreversible damage to the optic nerve head. Visual field loss, the functional change seen in glaucoma correlates well with structural loss in the neurosensory part of the eye involving the retinal ganglion cell layer (GCL) and retinal nerve fibre layer (RNFL). Early assessment and prevention of disease progression safeguard against visual field loss. Structural loss is evaluated via progressive stereoscopic optic disc photography and optical coherence tomography (OCT), which measures the GCL and RNFL thickness. Meanwhile, defects in visual fields indicate a functional loss. Ophthalmologists most correlate both the structural and functional data to interpret a patient's likelihood of glaucomatous damage and progression. In this chapter, we have elucidated means to correlate structural loss with functional loss in glaucoma patients from a neophyte's perspective and highlighted the finer nuances of these parameters in detail. This understanding of various terminologies related to structural and functional vision loss, along with the correlative interpretation of the structural and functional tests in a glaucoma patient, form the fulcrum of this chapter.

Keywords: Glaucoma, Structure-Function Correlation, Three-Dimensional, POAG, Optical Coherence Tomography, Visual Fields, Scanning Laser Ophthalmoscope, BMO-MRW

1. Introduction

Glaucoma is the upheaval in the structural and functional integrity of the optic nerve, whose progression can be arrested with judicious control of the intraocular pressure [1]. It includes a group of disorders characterised by chronic and progressive optic neuropathies. They exhibit characteristic morphological features at the optic nerve head and retinal nerve fibre layer which are associated with progressive loss of retinal ganglion cells leading to characteristic visual field defects [2]. Glaucoma is identified to be the leading cause of irreversible blindness on a global scale. The global prevalence among those aged 40 years and above has been estimated to be about 76 million in 2020. It is expected to keep rising to over 118 million affected patients by the year 2040. The disease shows a preference pattern for males, in comparison to females. People of African ancestry and people living in urban areas were more likely to be diagnosed with the disease than their counterparts of European ancestry and people living in rural areas [3]. The most common subtype among this group is primary open-angle glaucoma (POAG) [4]. POAG is distinctly regarded as a multi-factorial optic neuropathy. The typical pathology involved is the acquired atrophy of the optic nerve and loss of retinal ganglion cells in the background of open anterior chamber angles, giving rise to specific visual field disturbances [5–8]. The level of structural alteration, correlated with functional perception, is used to assess the severity of POAG among patients. Structural alterations encompass changes involving, but not limited to, neuro-retinal rim thinning and retinal nerve fibre layer loss (RNFL). Functional alteration in POAG can indicate a change in the visual function, most commonly, a visual field loss [9]. Measurements of these structural and functional components show a wide range of variation between patients and between repeated measurements on the same patient, making this a considerable challenge to assess the true extent of glaucomatous damage [9]. In day-to-day practice, in glaucoma clinics, this is overcome by using the structural domain to support the diagnosis, made using the functional domain and vice versa.

The Structural and functional integrals of glaucoma show a progressive decline as the disease progresses [10]. This decline shares a common pathophysiological pathway, which includes the death of the retinal ganglion cells and their axons, thereby alluding to the possibility of a defined relationship between these two integrals. Hence, establishing this relationship between structural and functional pathology of glaucoma, and their clinical measurements, gain weight in the practice of glaucoma management [11].

2. Importance of the structure: Function relationship in glaucoma

Delving into both the structural and functional progression of glaucoma, particularly in cases of POAG, while ascertaining the natural history of the disease to grade its severity is vital. These factors dictate and influence the course of treatment, as well as the visual prognosis of said patients.

The natural history of POAG includes progressive loss of the neuro-retinal rim width on the structural front coupled with progressive loss of the visual field on the functional front [12]. In a subset of patients, it was found that blindness was an imminent problem, whose risk depended on the severity of the disease at initial presentation [13].

However, in the grading of the severity, clinical dilemmas arise when there are discrepancies between the structural and functional presentation of the disease in the same patient. For instance, some patients who show end-stage glaucomatous optic atrophy do not show an equivalent representative severity of visual field loss. On the other end of the spectrum, patients with visual field loss characteristic of severe glaucoma do not show comparable structural defects [14, 15]. Such differences pose a diagnostic predicament to a glaucoma clinician on whether to base or judge the likelihood of the disease and severity on one component over the other, or a combination of both.

3. Evolution of fundus photography

The first historical fundus photograph dates back to 1886, published by Jackman and Webster [15]. However, the major limitation of this technique was a prominent corneal reflex, resulting in poor image clarity. By 1898, Thorner designed the first reflex-free ophthalmoscope based on a simple principle of viewing the transmitted and reflected beams through either half of a dilated pupil [16]. In the following year, Friedrich Dimmer further developed a relatively more complex ophthalmoscope in partnership with Zeiss Jena. Though a significant leap forward, this ophthalmoscope was large, hefty, and significantly more expensive [17, 18]. By 1925, the Zeiss-Nordensen retinal camera, which used a carbon arc lamp for imaging, was commercially made available. The Zeiss Littmann ophthalmoscope, invented in 1955 with an improved optical design and electronic flash illumination, ushered in a new era of fundus photography.

3.1 Scanning laser ophthalmoscope

The inception of the first scanner laser ophthalmoscope opened a third door in fundus photography. Designed by Webb, Hughes and Pomerantzeff, it required substantially less light than conventional ophthalmoscopes or fundus cameras. A laser beam of <100 μW provided a flying spot on the subject's retina, allowing an inversion of the usual division of the pupil; only the central half-millimetre is required for illumination, while the remaining area is used for light collection. No optical image of the retina is formed, but a photomultiplier tube in a pupillary conjugate plane provides video signals to a TV monitor, displaying an image.

The natural evolution of this scanning laser ophthalmoscope has undergone many iterations since. The field of view has expanded to wide-field and ultrawide-field imaging, which encompass nearly 200° of the retina (**Figure 1**). Confocal imaging, using blue, red, red-free and infrared spectrum imaging, help visualise the retinal architecture more clearly (**Figures 2** and **3**). Autofluorescence enables the assessment of the retinal pigment epithelial (RPE) layer integrity (**Figure 3**). Non-mydriatic cameras allow fundus and stereoscopic disc imaging in angle closure suspects (**Figure 4**) [19]. Red-free filtering enhances the visualisation of retinal vasculature. Blue images provide an improved view of the retinal nerve fibre layer (RNFL). The red channel allows it to penetrate the deeper layers of the choroid. Infrared light provides detailed information corresponding to the choroid.

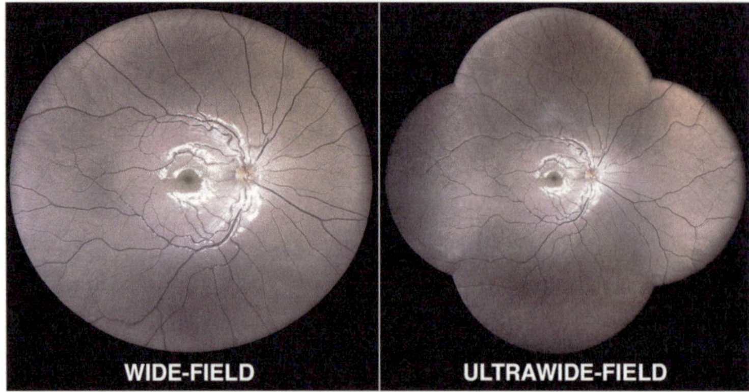

Figure 1.
Fundus photograph showing wide-field and ultrawide-field images of the same patient.

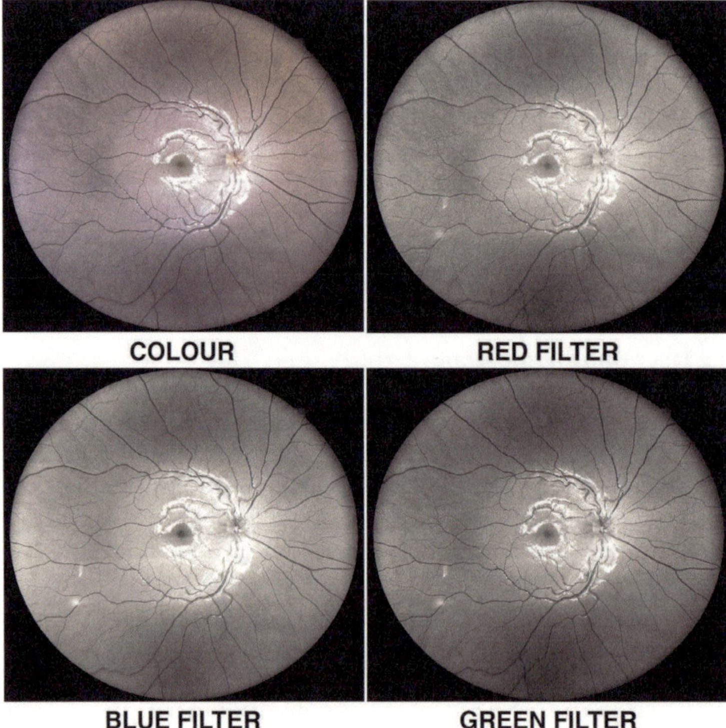

Figure 2.
Fundus photograph showing colour, red filter, blue filter & green filter images of the same patient.

4. Evolution of optical coherence tomography

Optical coherence tomography (OCT) was considered to enhance the low-coherence interferometry used initially for axial length measurements [19]. The initial systems were limited to scanning speeds of 400 axial scans (A-scans) because of a physical constraint: a moving reference mirror. Changing the position of the reference

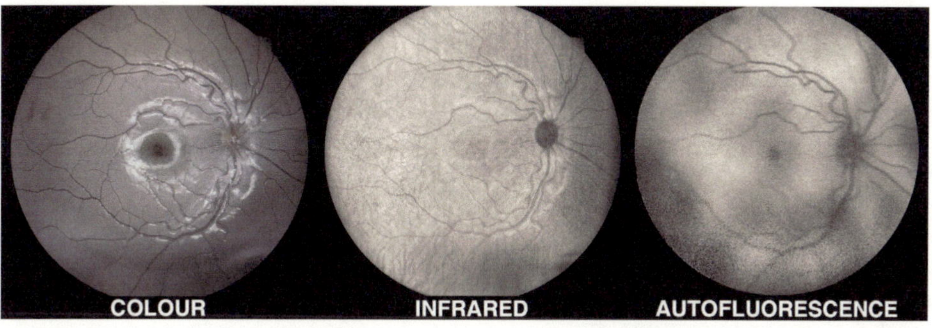

Figure 3.
Fundus photograph showing single field colour, infrared and autofluorescence image of the same patient.

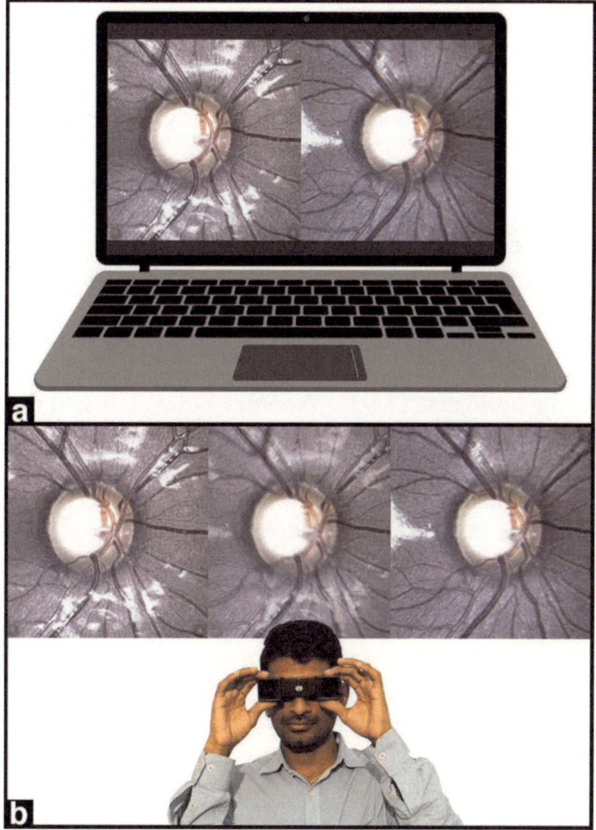

Figure 4
(a) Image showing the stereoscopic image of the right eye optic disc obtained through the fundus machine. (b) Image showing the observers' view of the stereoscopic image after wearing the 3D glasses.

mirror enabled backscattered tissue intensity levels from varying retinal and choroidal depths to be interpreted. The two main advancements incorporated into recent commercial systems are better axial resolution and increased scanning speeds [20–23]. The axial resolution was improved from 10 μ to 2 μ by incorporating broad-band light sources into the OCT systems [22]. Image acquisition speed has also been considerably improved through enhanced detection of backscattering signals without the need for movement of the reference mirror. Frequency information is acquired with either a broad-bandwidth light source, a charge-coupled device camera, and a spectrometer or by sweeping a narrow-bandwidth source through a broad range of frequencies with a photodetector [22–28]. Spectral-domain OCT (SD-OCT) uses broadband light sources while the swept source uses a narrow bandwidth through a broad range of frequencies.

Since its inception, OCT has seen numerous advances both in image acquisition capabilities as well as image recognition abilities. Adaptive optics OCT (AO-OCT) was introduced by Miller et al. in 2003 to improve transverse resolution [29]. Adaptive optics mainly compensate for monochromatic aberrations using wavefront sensing and deformable mirrors [30]. Ultrahigh (axial)-resolution AO-OCT was introduced in 2004, improving transverse resolution to 5 to 10 μm in the retina [31]. Polarisation-sensitive OCT detects polarisation changes in polarised light to detect lesions at the level of retinal pigment epithelium layer [32]. RNFL birefringence was measured in humans by Cense et al. and Yamanari et al. who found that, unlike RNFL thickness, birefringence does not change as a function of increasing radius from the ONH [33–35]. This is likely to play a role in better OCT image acquisition, going forward. Intraoperative OCT incorporates a 1310 nm imaging system coupled to an operating microsystem [36].

5. Evolution of visual fields

During the 5th century BC, Hippocrates observed and described hemianopia. Ptolemy attributed the visual field to be circular. Ulmus first published the first illustration of visual fields in 1602. Marriott described the blind spot for the first time with its relation to the optic disc [37–39]. Thomas Young labelled the extent of the visual field as 50° superiorly, 70° inferiorly, 60° nasally, and 90° temporally [37–39]. Non-seeing areas in the visual field were reported by Boerhaave in 1708, while Beer described the shape and location of scotomas in 1817. However, quantitative visual fields were only obtained in 1856, by Von Graefe.

Jannik Bjerrum introduced campimetry with the help of a tangent screen and, along with his assistant Henning Ronne, used different target sizes to generate multiple isopters to characterise the shape and three-dimensional characteristics of the visual field sensitivity map. In this regard, the most significant contribution was the invention of the Ganzfeld bowl perimetry by Goldmann in 1945, which provided a uniform dark background superimposed with a moving optical projection system [37–39]. Tubingher perimetry was invented by Elfried Aulhorn and Heinrich Harms, which essentially was a static perimeter capable of making temporal and spatial summations throughout the visual field. The problem with bowl perimetry was the development of artefacts related to masks and increased risks of infection. In the cases of Humphrey visual field progression cannot be overlooked. In 1974, Franz Frankhauser and co-workers developed the first automated perimeter, the Octopus [40–47].

Built-in automated tools to describe and analyse progression in the Octopus perimeter, provide the greatest advantages today (**Figure 5**). These include:

Global trend analysis: consists of four indices. They are mean defect, square root loss of variance, local defect and diffuse defect.

Cluster trend analysis: mainly evaluates the ganglion cell loss along the retinal nerve fibre layer and papillomacular bundle.

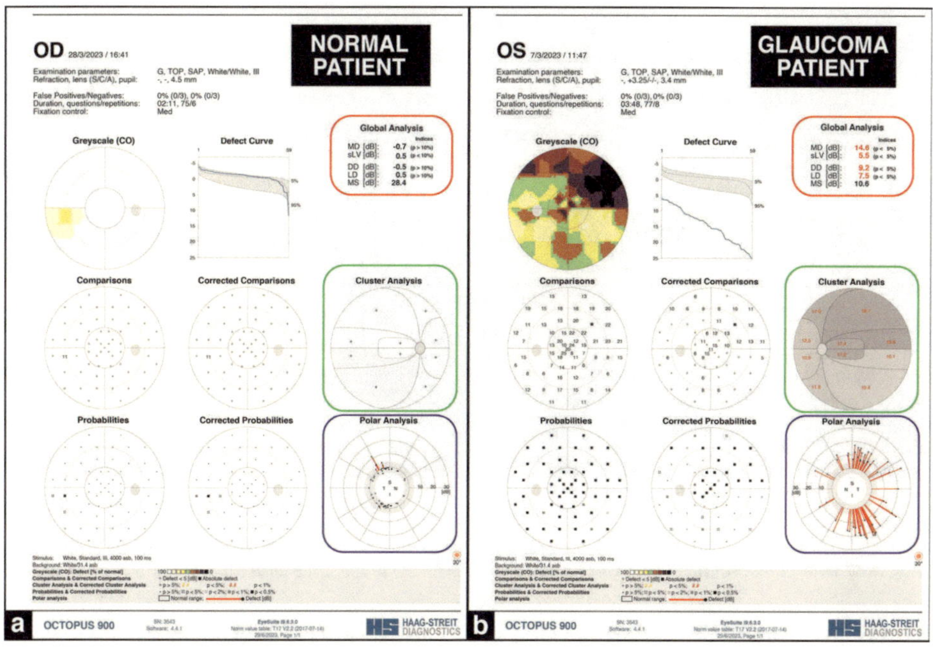

Figure 5.
(a) Visual field report of a normal patient showing the global trend analysis (red box), cluster trend analysis (green box) and polar trend analysis (blue box). (b) Visual field report of a glaucoma patient showing the global trend analysis (red box), cluster trend analysis (green box) and polar trend analysis (blue box).

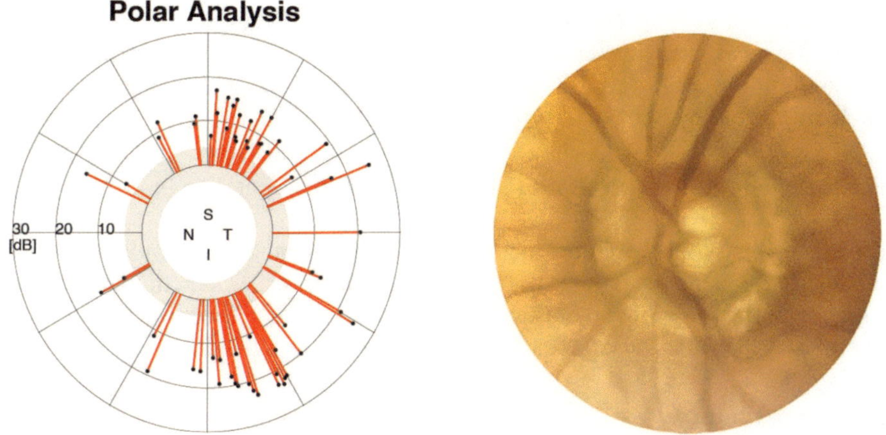

Figure 6.
Polar trend analysis (structural) correlated with the inferotemporal notching (functional) in the optic disc.

Polar trend analysis: aids in detecting the precise location of structural defects corresponding to the functional loss that has occurred (**Figure 6**).

5.1 Short-wavelength automated perimetry (SWAP)

The colour perimeter was introduced by Hart et al., which used iso-luminant blue and yellow light, and was later termed short-wavelength automated perimetry (SWAP). It

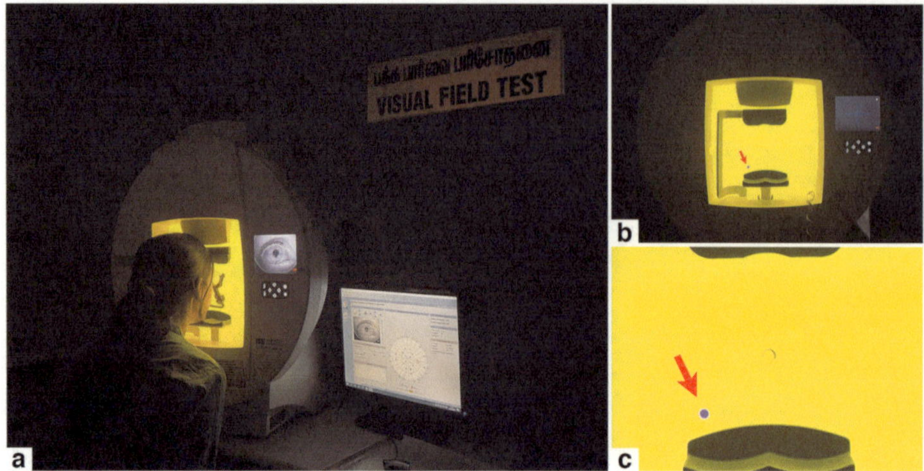

Figure 7.
(a) Image showing the patient performing the SITA SWAP perimetry. (b) Image demonstrating the yellow background with blue stimulus (red arrow) and (c) zoomed view of the same with blue stimulus (red arrow).

incorporates a bright yellow background to desensitise the red and green wavelengths, thus utilizing the shorter blue wavelength as a stimulus (**Figure** 7) [48–52].

5.2 Flicker perimetry

Flicker perimetry is based on an intermittent flashing stimulus superimposed on a uniform background [48]. Three types of tests based on flicker perimetry aim to detect the highest rate of flicker at higher contrast, the amplitude of contrast to detect flicker, and luminance pedestal flicker. The greatest advantage of flicker perimetry is that it is unaffected by blur.

5.3 Frequency doubling threshold (FDT) perimetry

Frequency doubling perimetry incorporates a sinusoidal grating under low spatial frequency that undergoes high temporal frequency counter-flicker, thus providing double the number of light and darker bars - a frequency-doubling effect. This form of perimetry is resistant to variations occurring in the environment.

5.4 Motion perimetry

Motion perimetry is based on motion sensitivity, which is a very primitive visual function and is resistant to change in many different stimuli.

Motion perimetry is based on [48, 53].

- Determining the minimum amount of movement needed for the detection of change in position - displacement perimetry
- Evaluating the amount of motion coherence needed to detect a direction of motion from within a group of randomly moving dots - motion coherence perimetry

- Determining the direction of motion
- Assessing the velocity needed for motion detection
- Measuring the size of a number of moving dots needed to localise the direction of motion

5.5 High-pass resolution perimetry

High-pass resolution perimetry employs light and dark concentric rings, from which low spatial frequency components have been removed to emphasize the lighter and darker edges. The main aim of high-pass resolution perimetry is to elevate the detection threshold so that the detection and identification thresholds coincide simultaneously [54].

5.6 Rarebit perimetry

Very small stimuli are displayed on a video display, where 0, 1, or 2 suprathreshold stimuli are presented at different local visual field regions. The number of dots the patient was able to appreciate was then noted [55, 56].

6. The amalgamation of the three musketeers - the Spectralis, the Octopus and the EIDON

While examining the posterior pole, primarily for structural evaluation, we observe the scleral rim to determine the margin of the optic disc. However, in reality, the margins are defined by Bruch's membrane opening (BMO), which is an OCT interpretation. The Bruch's membrane opening-minimum rim width (BMO-MRW) (**Figure 8**) is a superior parameter for assessing the progression of glaucomatous damage, significantly outperforming Bruch's membrane opening horizontal rim width (BMO-HRW) [57].

Additionally, the position of the fovea may vary as a result of torsional movements of the patient's eye, potentially leading to erroneous results [58–62]. The Spectralis

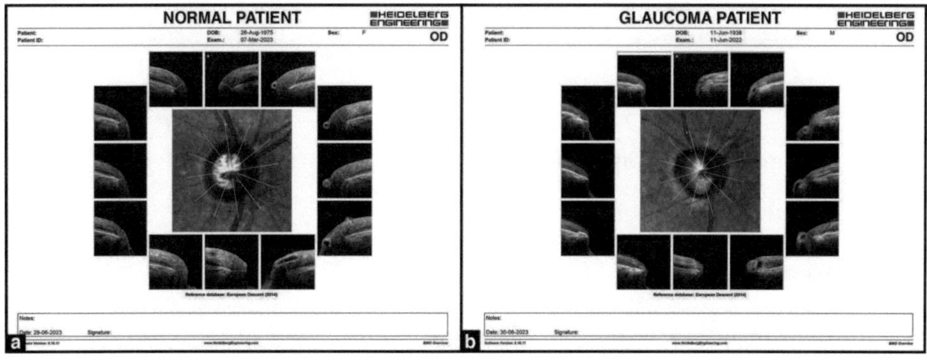

Figure 8.
(a) Image showing the Bruch's membrane—minimum rim width analysis in Spectralis OCT of a normal patient. (b) Image showing the Bruch's membrane—minimum rim width (reduced) analysis in Spectralis OCT of a glaucoma patient.

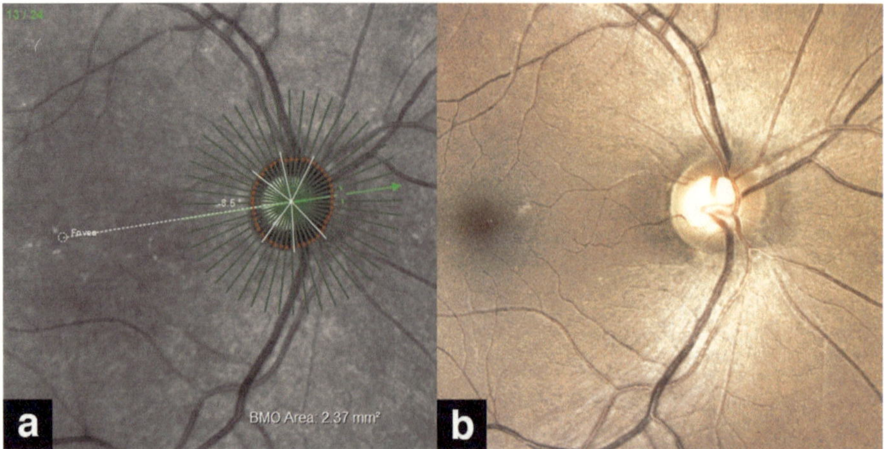

Figure 9.
(a) Fovea Bruch's membrane opening axis (FoBMO) measured using the anatomical positioning system. (b) Fundus image of the same showing the fovea.

OCT incorporates an anatomical positioning system technique for precise marking of the fovea Bruch's membrane opening axis (FoBMO) (**Figure 9**). This process includes marking the centre of the fovea and BMO-MRW, formation of the FoBMO axis, and analyzing parameters related to it. This approach effectively eliminates errors resulting from torsional eye movements.

BMO MRW components:

- Black line: Measured BMO MRW
- Grey curve: Baseline values
- Horizontal axis: Position along optic disc circumference in degrees

Confocal scanning laser ophthalmoscope uses three display options:

- BMO points and section images
- BMO display points
- OCT section image

The functional correlation of the BMO-MRW is compared with the polar analysis of the OCTOPUS perimeter.

6.1 Polar trend analysis

Polar trend analysis assesses the point-wise trend analysis of the sensitivity loss in decibels, instead of a slope method to determine the rate of change. Sensitivity loss for the first visual field is represented as blue, while the last field is depicted as yellow. These two points are based on the trend lines, not the individual visual fields on that day. The two sensitivity lines are then plotted on a polar grid and are connected by a straight line corresponding to the position of nerve fibre bundles of the test location. If there is a worsening in sensitivity between the first and last points, then it is represented as a red bar. Improvement is depicted as a green bar. The grey band in the centre indicates the normal range for these bars.

- Location of the bar indicates a corresponding structural area
- Length of the bar denotes the amount of sensitivity loss in dB
- Longer bars denote the greater magnitude of the effect
- Colour of the bar is red – loss of sensitivity
- Colour of the bar is green – a gain of sensitivity

6.2 Cluster trend analysis

In Cluster trend analysis, visual field locations corresponding to the same RNFL bundle are grouped in 10 visual field clusters and used to calculate the respective average Cluster Mean Defect.

- Highly likely normal clusters (P > 5%) are marked with a "+" symbol, and are likely abnormal
- Cluster Mean defects are displayed in normal font (P < 5%) or bold font (P < 1%).
- The Corrected Cluster Analysis representation is similar, but eliminates diffuse visual field loss and solely considers local loss.

RNFL thickness measured clinically by fundus examination and true colour confocal fundus imaging (EIDON) is correlated with RNFL analysis of Spectralis OCT, which is then functionally correlated with cluster analysis of the Octopus perimeter (**Figure 10**). Similarly, the papillomacular bundle

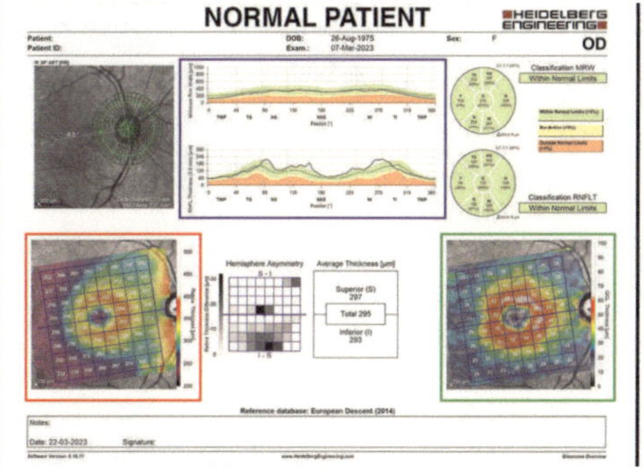

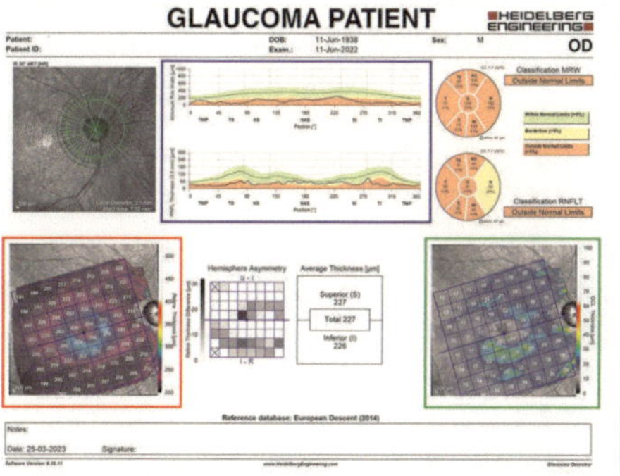

Figure 10.
OCT RNFL reports of a normal and glaucoma patient respectively with RNFL thickness (red box), GCL thickness (green box), BMO-MRW and RNFL thickness comparative analysis map (blue box).

examined clinically will be correlated with the macular ganglion cell inner plexiform layer analysis of Spectralis OCT (**Figure 10**).

7. Conclusion

It is important to do a structure-function correlation to continuously monitor glaucoma progression. The structure-function correlation of optic disc analysis involves stereoscopic optic disc photography, polar analysis and BMO-MRW determination (**Figure 11**); RNFL analysis involves OCT-RNFL and 24-2 visual field analysis (**Figure 12**); GCL analysis involves OCT (GCL, Inner Plexiform Layer and facultative mRNFL), 24-2 and 10-2 visual field analysis (**Figure 13**) [63]. Each aspect of the disease can be monitored with a 3-D approach in imaging and analysis.

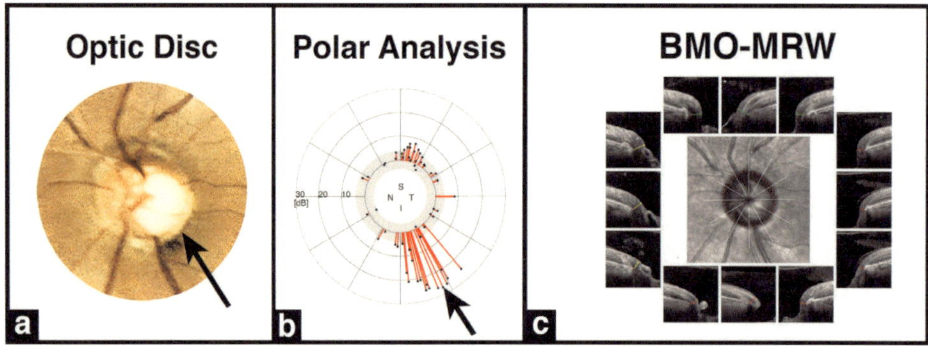

Figure 11.
Image showing (a) inferior notching (black arrow) in the optic disc. (b) Corresponding inferior defect in the polar analysis map (black arrow). (c) Bruch's membrane—minimum rim width analysis in Spectralis OCT showing inferior defect.

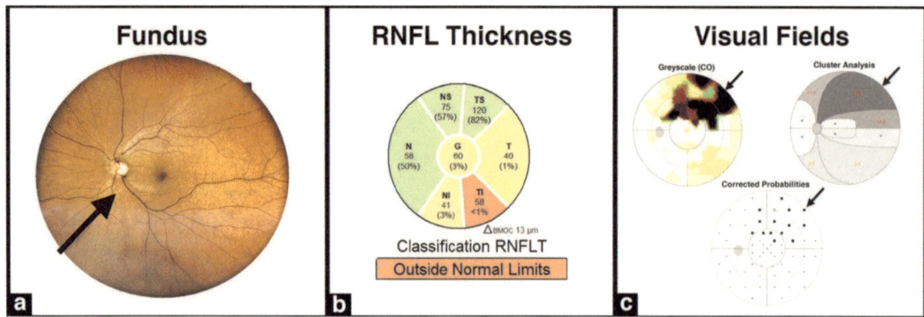

Figure 12.
(a) Fundus photograph showing inferior RNFL wedge defect (black arrow). (b) RNFL thickness map showing inferotemporal thinning. (c) Visual field evaluation (greyscale, cluster analysis and corrected probabilities) showing superior visual field defect (black arrows).

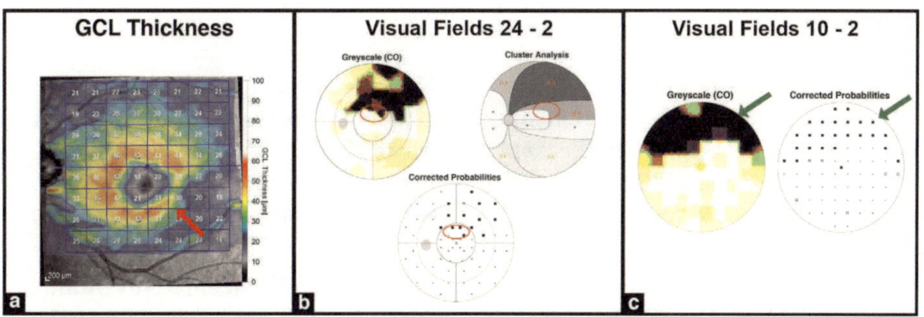

Figure 13.
(a) GCL thickness map showing inferior thinning of the ganglion cell layer (red arrow). (b) Visual field 24-2 evaluation (greyscale, cluster analysis and corrected probabilities) showing the corresponding visual field defect in the central 10 degrees of field (red circles). (c) Corresponding functional damage easily detected in visual field 10-2 (greyscale and corrected probabilities) evaluation (green arrows).

Author details

Prasanna Venkatesh Ramesh[1*], Anujeet Paul[2], Shruthy Vaishali Ramesh[3], Niranjan Karthik Senthil Kumar[4], Prajnya Ray[5], Aji Kunnath Devadas[5], Navaneeth Krishna[5], Meena Kumari Ramesh[3] and Ramesh Rajasekaran[6]

1 Department of Glaucoma and Research, Mahathma Eye Hospital Private Limited, Trichy, Tamil Nadu, India

2 Department of Vitreo-Retina, B.B. Eye Foundation, Kolkata, West Bengal, India

3 Department of Cataract and Refractive Surgery, Mahathma Eye Hospital Private Limited, Trichy, Tamil Nadu, India

4 Department of Comprehensive Ophthalmology, Nirmal Eye Hospital, Chennai, Tamil Nadu, India

5 Department of Optometry and Visual Science, Mahathma Eye Hospital Private Limited, Trichy, Tamil Nadu, India

6 Department of Paediatric Ophthalmology and Strabismus, Mahathma Eye Hospital Private Limited, Trichy, Tamil Nadu, India

*Address all correspondence to: email2prajann@gmail.com

References

[1] Stamper RL, Lieberman MF, Drake MV. Chapter 1, introduction and classification of Glaucomas. In: Becker-Shaffer's Diagnosis and Therapy of the Glaucomas. 8th ed. Edinburgh: Mosby, Elsevier; 2009. pp. 1-2

[2] European Glaucoma Society. Terminology and Guidelines for Glaucoma. 3rd ed. Savona: Editrice Dogma; 2008. Italy Editrice Dogma. p. 2008

[3] Tham YC, Li X, Wong TY, Quigley HA, Aung T, Cheng CY. Global prevalence of glaucoma and projections of glaucoma burden through 2040: A systematic review and meta-analysis. Ophthalmology. 2014;**121**(11):2081-2090

[4] Lee DA, Higginbotham EJ. Glaucoma and its treatment: A review. American Journal of Health-System Pharmacy. 2005;**62**(7):691-699

[5] Prum BE, Rosenberg LF, Gedde SJ, Mansberger SL, Stein JD, Moroi SE, et al. Primary open-angle glaucoma preferred practice pattern® guidelines. Ophthalmology. 2016;**123**(1):P41-P111

[6] Ramesh PV, K A, Ray P, Ramesh SV, Ramesh MK, Rajasekaran R, et al. Combating anti-glaucoma medication compliance issues among literate urban Indian population-has this fallen in our blind spot? Journal of Clinical Ophthalmology. 2021;**5**(S5):1-472-47

[7] Ramesh PV, Ray P, Senthil NK, Ramesh SV, Devadas AK. Commentary: Minimally invasive glaucoma surgery for a surgical take diversion: An economic perspective. Indian Journal of Ophthalmology. 2023;**71**(2):566-568

[8] Keltner JL, Johnson CA, Anderson DR, Levine RA, Fan J, Cello KE, et al. The association between glaucomatous visual fields and optic nerve head features in the ocular hypertension treatment study. Ophthalmology. 2006;**113**(9):1603-1612

[9] European Glaucoma Prevention Study (EGPS) Group. Results of the European glaucoma prevention study. Ophthalmology. 2005;**112**(3):366-375

[10] Read RM, Spaeth GL. The practical clinical appraisal of the optic disc in glaucoma: The natural history of cup progression and some specific disc-field correlations. American Academy of Ophthalmology and Otolaryngology. 1974;**78**(2):OP255-274

[11] Ramesh PV, Ramesh SV, Ray P, Devadas AK. Commentary: The never-ending story of COVID-19: Accustoming to the new abnormal in glaucoma practice. Indian Journal of Ophthalmology. 2023 Mar;**71**(3):868

[12] AGIS investigators. The advanced glaucoma intervention study (AGIS): Comparison of treatment outcomes within race: 10-year results. Ophthalmology. 2004;**111**(4):651-664

[13] Grant WM, Burke JF. Why do some people go blind from glaucoma? Ophthalmology. 1982;**89**(9):991-998

[14] Malik R, Swanson WH, Garway-Heath DF. "Structure-function relationship" in glaucoma: Past thinking and current concepts. Clinical & Experimental Ophthalmology. 2012; **40**(4):369-380

[15] Jackman WT, Webster JD. On photographing the retina of the living eye. Philadelphia Photographer. 1886;**23**: 340-341 Available from: http://www.a

rchive.org/stream/philadelphiaph ot18861phil#page/340/mode/1up

[16] Thorner W. A new stationary ophthalmoscope without reflexes. American Journal of Ophthalmology. 1899;**16**:330-345

[17] Die DF. Photographie des Augenhintergrundes. Weisbaden: Bergmann; 1907. p. 1907 Available from: http://archive.org/details/diephotographied00dimm

[18] Ramesh PV, Ray P, Joshua T, Devadas AK, Raj PM, Ramesh SV, et al. The photoreal new-age innovative pedagogical & counseling tool for glaucoma with 3D augmented reality (eye MG AR). European Journal of Ophthalmology. 2023;0(0)

[19] Ramesh PV, Parthasarthi S, Ramesh SV, Rajasekaran R, Ramesh MK. Interconnecting ophthalmic gadgets (infinity stones) at finger tips (personal computer desktop) with local area network for safe and effective practice during COVID-19 crises. Indian Journal of Ophthalmology. Feb 2021; **69**(2):449

[20] Drexler W, Morgner U, Kartner FX, et al. In vivo ultrahigh-resolution optical coherence tomography. Optics Letters. 1999;**24**:1221-1223

[21] Unterhuber A, Povazay B, Bizheva K, et al. Advances in broad bandwidth light sources for ultrahigh resolution optical coherence tomography. Physics in Medicine and Biology. 2004;**49**:1235-1246

[22] Wojtkowski M, Leitgeb R, Kowalczyk A, Bajraszewski T, Fercher A. In vivo human retinal imaging by Fourier-domain optical coherence tomography. Journal of Biomedical Optics. 2002;7:457-463

[23] Choma M, Sarunic M, Yang C, Izatt J. Sensitivity advantage of swept source and Fourier domain optical coherence tomography. Optics Express. 2003;**11**:2183-2189

[24] de Boer JF, Cense B, Park BH, Pierce MC, Tearney GJ, Bouma BE. Improved signal-to-noise ratio in spectral-domain compared with time-domain optical coherence tomography. Optics Letters. 2003;**28**:2067-2069

[25] Leitgeb R, Wojtkowski M, Kowalczyk A, Hitzenberger CK, Sticker M, Fercher AF. Spectral measurement of absorption by spectroscopic frequency-domain optical coherence tomography. Optics Letters. 2000;**25**:820-822

[26] Wojtkowski M, Srinivasan V, Fujimoto JG, et al. Three-dimensional retinal imaging with high-speed ultrahigh-resolution optical coherence tomography. Ophthalmology. 2005;**112**: 1734-1746

[27] Choma MA, Hsu K, Izatt JA. Swept source optical coherence tomography using an all-fiber 1300-nm ring laser source. Journal of Biomedical Optics. 2005;**10**:44009

[28] Zhang J, Rao B, Chen Z. Swept source based Fourier domain functional optical coherence tomography. Conference Proceedings: Annual International Conference of the IEEE Engineering in Medicine and Biology Society. 2005;7:7230-7233

[29] Miller DT, Qu J, Jonnal RS, Thorn KE. Coherence gating and adaptive optics in the eye. 2003;**4956**:65-72. Available from: https://ui.adsabs.harvard.edu/abs/2003SPIE.4956...65M

[30] Babcock HW. The possibility of compensating astronomical seeing.

Publications of the Astronomical Society of the Pacific. 1953;**65**:229-236

[31] Hermann B, Fernandez EJ, Unterhuber A, et al. Adaptive-optics ultrahigh-resolution optical coherence tomography. Optics Letters. 2004;**29**: 2142-2144

[32] de Boer JF, Milner TE, van Gemert MJ, Nelson JS. Two-dimensional birefringence imaging in biological tissue by polarization-sensitive optical coherence tomography. Optics Letters. 1997;**22**:934-936

[33] Cense B, Chen TC, Park BH, Pierce MC, de Boer JF. In vivo birefringence and thickness measurements of the human retinal nerve fiber layer using polarization-sensitive optical coherence tomography. Journal of Biomedical Optics. 2004;**9**:121-125

[34] Cense B, Chen TC, Park BH, Pierce MC, de Boer JF. Thickness and birefringence of healthy retinal nerve fiber layer tissue measured with polarization-sensitive optical coherence tomography. Investigative Ophthalmology & Visual Science. 2004; **45**:2606-2612

[35] Yamanari M, Miura M, Makita S, Yatagai T, Yasuno Y. Phase retardation measurement of retinal nerve fiber layer by polarization-sensitive spectral-domain optical coherence tomography and scanning laser polarimetry. Journal of Biomedical Optics. 2008;**13**:014013

[36] Geerling G, Muller M, Winter C, et al. Intraoperative 2-dimensional optical coherence tomography as a new tool for anterior segment surgery. Archives of Ophthalmology. 2005;**123**: 253-257

[37] Johnson C, Wall M, Thompson H. A history of perimetry and visual field testing. Optometry and Vision Science: Official Publication of the American Academy of Optometry. 2011;**88**:E8-15

[38] Lascaratos J, Marketos S. A historical outline of Greek ophthalmology from the Hellenistic period up to the establishment of the first universities. Documenta Ophthalmologica. 1988;**68**: 157-169

[39] Thompson HS. How visual field testing was introduced into office ophthalmology. In: David G, editor. Cogan Ophthalmic Historical Society Meeting. 1993

[40] Bebie H, Fankhauser F, Spahr J. Static perimetry: Strategies. Acta Ophthalmologica. 1976;**54**:325-338

[41] Bebie H, Fankhauser F, Spahr J. Static perimetry: Accuracy and fluctuations. Acta Ophthalmologica. 1976;**54**:339-348

[42] Fankhauser F, Spahr J, Bebie H. Three years of experience with the 'Octopus' automatic perimeter. Documenta Ophthalmologica Proceedings Series. 1977;**14**:7-15

[43] Ramesh P, Vaishali R, Ray P, Kunnath A, Ramesh M, Rajasekaran R. The curious cases of incorrect face mask positions in bowl-type perimetry versus enclosed chamber perimetry during the COVID-19 pandemic. Indian Journal of Ophthalmology. 2021;**69**:2236-2239

[44] Ramesh PV, Devadas AK, Senthil NK, Sainath D. Commentary: Rethinking 10-2 visual fields in early diagnosis of glaucoma for a glided glaucoma practice: The right choice to pick up a feeble noise? Indian Journal of Ophthalmology. 2023;**71**(3):860-863

[45] Ramesh PV, Devadas AK, Ramesh SV, Sainath D. Commentary: An

ode to the perimetrist with novel strategies for priming the patient before the psychophysical subjective perimetry test. Indian Journal of Ophthalmology. 2023;**71**(2):574-575

[46] Fankhauser F. Developmental milestones of automated perimetry. In: Hendkind P, editor. ACTA: XXIV International Congress of Ophthalmology. Philadelphia, PA: JB Lippincott; 1982. pp. 147-150

[47] Hart WM Jr, Hartz RK, Hagen RW, Clark KW. Color contrast perimetry. Investigative Ophthalmology & Visual Science. 1984;**25**:400-413

[48] Johnson CA, Sample PA. Perimetry and visual field testing. In: Alm A, Kaufmann P, editors. Adler's Physiology of the Eye: Clinical Approach. 10th ed. St. Louis, MO: Mosby; 2002. pp. 552-577

[49] Demirel S, Johnson CA. Short wavelength automated perimetry (SWAP) in ophthalmic practice. Journal of the American Optometric Association. 1996;**67**:451-456

[50] Johnson CA. Diagnostic value of short-wavelength automated perimetry. Current Opinion in Ophthalmology. 1996;7:54-58

[51] Sample PA. Short-wavelength automated perimetry: it's role in the clinic and for understanding ganglion cell function. Progress in Retinal and Eye Research. 2000;**19**:369-383

[52] Racette L, Sample PA. Short-wavelength automated perimetry. Ophthalmology Clinics of North America. 2003;**16**:227-236 vi–vii

[53] Wall M, Ketoff KM. Random dot motion perimetry in glaucoma patients and normal subjects. American Journal of Ophthalmology. 1995;**120**:587-596

[54] Keltner JL, Johnson CA. Comparative material on automated and semiautomated perimeters—1986. Ophthalmology. 1986;**93**:1-25

[55] Frise'n L. New, sensitive window on abnormal spatial vision: Rarebit probing. Vision Research. 2002;**42**:1931-1939

[56] Brusini P, Salvetat ML, Parisi L, Zeppieri M. Probing glaucoma visual damage by rarebit perimetry. The British Journal of Ophthalmology. 2005;**89**: 180-184

[57] Ramesh PV, Ramesh SV, Ramesh MK, Rajasekaran R, Parthasarathi S. Striking the metronome in morphometric analysis of glaucoma - shifting from Bruch's membrane opening - horizontal rim width (BMO-HRW) to Bruch's membrane opening - minimum rim width (BMO-MRW). Indian Journal of Ophthalmology. 2021;**69**:1005-1008

[58] Ramesh P, Subramaniam T, Ray P, Devadas A, Vaishali R, Ansar S, et al. Utilizing human intelligence in artificial intelligence for detecting glaucomatous fundus images using human-in-the-loop machine learning. Indian Journal of Ophthalmology. 2022;**70**:1131-1138

[59] Ramesh PV, Ramesh SV, Aji K, Ray P, Tamilselvan S, Parthasarathi S, et al. Modeling and mitigating human annotations to design processing systems with human-in-the-loop machine learning for glaucomatous defects: The future in artificial intelligence. Indian Journal of Ophthalmology. 2021;**69**(10):2892-2894

[60] Ramesh PV, Ramesh SV, Devadas AK, Ramesh MK, Rajasekaran R. Response to comments on: Modeling and mitigating human annotations to design processing systems with human-in-the-loop machine learning for glaucomatous defects: The future in artificial intelligence. Indian Journal of Ophthalmology. 2022;**8670**(8):316461

[61] Ramesh PV, Parthasarathi S, Ramesh SV, Devadas AK, Ray P, Rajasekaran R. Decoding glaucoma module premium edition. Indian Journal of Ophthalmology 2022;**70**(6):2211

[62] Ramesh PV, Panneerselvan P, Devadas AK. Pick up early glaucoma: unveiling the blind truth with the 10-2 visual field. Haryana Journal of Ophthalmology. 2023;**XV**(1)

[63] Ramesh PV, Devadas AK, Varsha V, Mohanty B, Ray P, Balamurugan A, et al. A rare case of unilateral Axenfeld–Rieger anomaly associated with optic disc coloboma: A multimodal imaging canvas. Indian Journal of Ophthalmology. Jul 2022;**70**(7):2645

Chapter 3

Ab-Interno Canaloplasty and Ab-Interno Canaloplasty/Trabeculotomy in Glaucoma Patients Using the OMNI Surgical System

Karsten Klabe and Andreas Fricke

Abstract

Eyes with Primary Open Angle Glaucoma (POAG) show anatomical changes within the trabecular outflow tract that increase aqueous humor outflow resistance and thus Intraocular Pressure (IOP). In these glaucomatous eyes, approximately 50–70% of the total outflow resistance is attributed by changes in the tissue of the Trabecular Meshwork (TM) and 30–50% by changes in Schlemm's canal and/or the collector canals. In the last decade, a number of Minimally Invasive Glaucoma Surgeries (MIGS) have been developed to target the different tissue changes particularly. For example, goniotomy, trabeculotomy, and trans-TM implants target TM resistance, whereas canaloplasty, viscodilation, and stenting procedures target Schlemm's canal and collector channels. Therefore, a procedure targeting multiple pathways of aqueous humor outflow might be more effective in lowering IOP. In a limited number of studies to date using the OMNI Surgical System either combined with phacoemulsification or as standalone system, IOP reductions of 20–35% and medication reductions of 25–75% have been reported. In this chapter, the experience in performing canaloplasty/trabeculotomy of Schlemm's canal and distal collector channels using the OMNI Surgical System is described.

Keywords: primary open-angle glaucoma, canaloplasty, trabeculotomy, OMNI Surgical System, glaucoma patients

1. Introduction

Glaucoma is still the second leading cause of blindness. The most important risk factors for glaucoma-related blindness are the severity of the disease at diagnosis, bilateral disease, and age. Currently, the only effective approach to preserving visual function in glaucoma is the reduction of the intraocular pressure (IOP) [1]. The first-line therapy for lowering intraocular pressure is usually the administration of medication in the form of eye drops. Poor compliance and tolerability can sometimes lead to treatment failure. For progressive glaucoma with surgical intervention, ab-externo filtration surgery is still considered the gold standard, but the procedure can lead to significant complications [2].

Within the last decade new surgical procedures have been established, which are summarized under the term Minimally Invasive Glaucoma Surgery (MIGS). MIGS have been developed as safer and less traumatic surgical interventions for patients with mild to moderate glaucoma or who are intolerant to standard medical therapy. They are characterized by an ab-interno approach, inducing minimal trauma and disruption of eye anatomy with conjunctiva sparing and a rapid recovery [3, 4]. These surgical procedures play an increasing role in the care of patients with mild to moderate glaucoma. To improve physiologic outflow, a variety of different glaucoma surgeries target the structures in the chamber angle.

The implementation of the therapeutic goal varies from patient to patient and requires the use of individual procedures to achieve maximum intraocular pressure reduction. Compared to trabeculectomy with the use of cytostatics, the achievable pressure reduction with MIGS is usually slightly lower. However, the major advantage of MIGS is the significantly improved intra- and postoperative complication rate. In addition, more individualized glaucoma therapy is possible due to the broad spectrum of MIGS procedures available today.

The OMNI Surgical System (Sight Science) is a single-handed device.

designed to introduce pre-dosed viscoelastic fluid into Schlemm's canal and incise trabecular meshwork tissue with a microcatheter. The device integrates an access cannula, a microcatheter, an internal fluid resorvoir, and a wheel mechanism for advancing and retracting the catheter. The device allows stretching of Schlemm's canal and trabeculotomy in the entire circumference (2 × 180°) by ab-interno technique with a single clear cornea incision [4]. This feasible combined surgery of trabeculotomy and viscodilation ab-interno was a new approach for which the device was developed and has been on the market since 2018 (original clearance Dec 21, 2017; updated August 11, 2020 and March 1, 2021) by the US Food and Medication Administration) [5].

1.1 Medical therapy and the problem of patient adherence to therapy

The target of currently available glaucoma medications is to preserve visual function by lowering intraocular pressure to prevent further damage to the optic nerve. Glaucoma is a chronic disease, so medication or non-medication therapy is a long-term treatment. This requires continuous and reliable cooperation of the patient (adherence). One of the difficulties of glaucoma is the asymptomatic nature of the disease in the early stages of the disease. Initial visual field defects are not yet perceived or they are compensated by the other eye. To improve patient adherence, persistence, and concordance, a high level of organization and motivation is required, both on the part of the physician and the patient. This is especially true when the patient does not directly perceive the effect of therapy due to the asymptomatic nature of glaucoma. The non-administration of medication leads to a stronger progression of glaucoma. Since overall adherence to medical therapy is rather poor, especially in glaucoma patients, good cooperation between physician and patient is beneficial for successful therapy. For example, a 2005 publication showed that only 50% of patients with newly diagnosed open-angle glaucoma attended immediate follow-up examinations. After 24 months, only 30% of patients adhered to the proposed medicinally treatment plan [6, 7].

Currently, there are a large number of publications describing a variety of problems and difficulties in taking glaucoma medications, these range from the number of medications to the drip mechanism to the affordability of the medications. Further publications deal with modern control mechanisms for adherence to the drip schedule (e.g., reminder via phone-app) [8–11]. In summary, a complicated treatment regimen with multiple different medications is counterproductive to increasing patient adherence; the simpler the treatment regimen, the more likely patients are to adhere to it. Surgical interventions such as MIGS are one way to reduce multiple medication administration.

1.2 Surgical interventions and minimally invasive glaucoma surgery (MIGS)

If medication treatment proves insufficient to achieve the targeted IOP or the drops are not well tolerated, laser or surgical treatment must be considered to prevent irreversible progression of the glaucomatous damage.

In the EGS guidelines [1], the indication for a glaucoma surgery is described as follows: Surgery should be considered whenever medical or laser treatment is unlikely to maintain sight in the glaucomatous eye. It should not be as a last resort. The indications for the different surgical techniques depend on the type of glaucoma, the target pressure, the medical history, the patients' risk profile, preferences and experience of the surgeon, and the patients' preference, expectation and postoperative adherence.

According to recommendations from Sweden and England, the use of surgical procedures may be considered as initial therapy or very early after initiation of medication therapy if the patient has a very high baseline pressure, early progression, persistent intolerance of medication alternatives, or apparent lack of compliance with therapy [7, 12].

Trabeculectomy is still considered the surgical gold standard, but it is not free of potentially serious complications. In addition, strict postoperative care is required to achieve clinically successful outcomes. To minimize the risks of conventional filtering surgery, MIGS have been developed as safer and less invasive techniques. Trabectome, approved in 2006, ushered in the new era of minimally invasive glaucoma surgery. Since then, a variety of MIGS devices and procedures have been developed and are currently available [4, 13–15].

The success of MIGS is significantly influenced by the preoperative conjunctival situation. Long-term drop application leads to a proven inflammation of the conjunctiva with an increase of lymphocytes, mast cells, and fibroblasts, among others. Therefore, it is recommended to discontinue local anti-glaucomatous drop therapy prior to surgery and allow regeneration of the ocular surface.

Most surgical procedures target the structures of physiologic aqueous humor outflow (trabecular meshwork, Schlemm's canal, collector channels) to lower IOP. Procedures fall into three categories:

a. Procedures that use stents to reduce outflow resistance (iStent, Hydrus microstent).

b. Procedures that cause viscodilation of Schlemm's canal and dilation of the trabecular meshwork (ab-interno canaloplasty, iTrack Advance, OMNI Surgical System).

c. Procedures that open or resect all or part of the trabecular meshwork (ab-interno trabeculotomy, Gonioscopy-Assisted Transluminal Trabeculotomy (GATT), OMNI Surgical System, ELIOS excimer laser trabeculotomy, high-frequency deep sclerotomy) [16].

Some MIGS, particularly implantable microstents, are approved for use in mild to moderate glaucoma at the time of cataract surgery. In patients with early glaucoma, cataract surgeons can perform a MIGS in the same surgical session as cataract surgery, knowing that they are associated with low-risk surgery and offer some benefit in lowering intraocular pressure beyond the benefit of lens extraction alone.

The patient's personal situation should also be considered when choosing the MIGS procedure. The usually reduced number of IOP-lowering medications after MIGS (compared to pre-surgery) often leads to a simpler treatment regimen and thus to better adherence to therapy and thus to an increased quality of life for the patient.

2. OMNI Surgical System: surgery procedure

Traditional canaloplasty procedures required an invasive ab-externo approach requiring full thickness scleral incisions. In many modern MIGS procedures, the surgery is performed through an ab-interno approach, thus there is significant protection of the conjunctiva and sclera.

The OMNI Surgical System (Sight Sciences, Inc., Menlo Park CA, USA) is indicated for catheterization and transluminal viscodilation of Schlemm's canal and incision into the trabecular meshwork to reduce intraocular pressure in adult patients with Open-Angle Glaucoma (OAG). The device should not be used in glaucoma patients in whom the chamber angle is compromised or damaged, nor in patients with chamber angle recession, neovascular glaucoma, chronic chamber angle closure, narrow-angle glaucoma, traumatic glaucoma, or malignant glaucoma.

The device allows repeated penetration of the Schlemm's canal with the microcatheter included. The surgeon gets the possibility to perform a complete 360° treatment or a partial treatment of less than 360° adapted to the medical needs of the patient. The system consists of a hand grip that opens into a curved cannula. The microcatheter is firmly integrated into the system, as is a reservoir that holds the viscoelastic (**Figure 1**). The surgical procedure itself has been well described in a number of previous publications [4, 5, 15, 17–20].

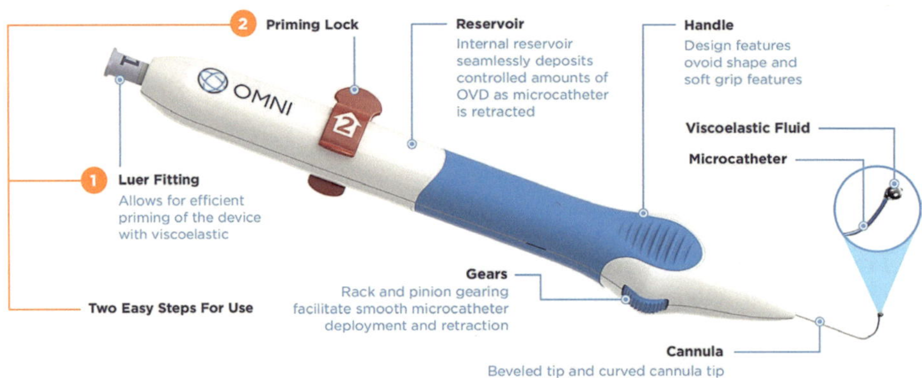

Figure 1.
OMNI Surgical System (figure used with permission from Sight Sciences, Inc. 2023).

2.1 Canaloplasty (viscodilation)

A small (1.5–2 mm) temporal free corneal incision is performed. After irrigation of the anterior chamber and deepening with viscoelastic, the head is tilted away from the surgeon and the microscope is tilted toward the surgeon for gonioscopic visualization (both approx. 30°–40°). The OMNI Surgical System is prepared by removing the retaining pin on the back of the handle and filling the reservoir with Healon. The cannula of the OMNI device is introduced through the incision into the anterior chamber and positioned at the desired location. Under gonioscopic view the cannula tip is brought near the nasal trabecular meshwork and a small <1 mm goniotomy was created. The microcatheter is then advanced into Schlemm's canal up to 180°. After then the microcatheter is slowly withdrawn while a fixed volume of approximately 11 μl of viscoelastic is automatically dispensed into Schlemm's canal and the collector channels. The procedure is then repeated for the second 180° of the canal. To avoid undesirable suprachoroidal tip advancement, the surgeon must ensure that the trabecular meshwork is penetrated at the correct location. The blue microcannula must be clearly visible in Schlemm's canal (**Figure 2**). Blood reflux indicates successful catheterization of Schlemm's canal. After the cannula is withdrawn from the eye, the anterior chamber is irrigated to entirely remove the Healon.

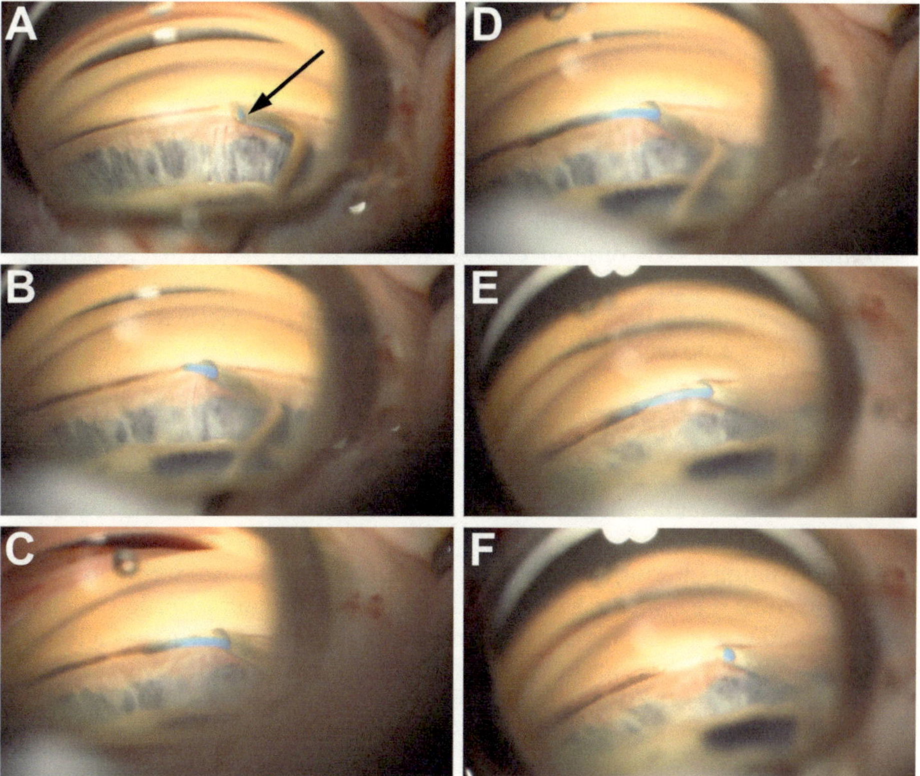

Figure 2.
Gonioscopic view of circumferential viscodilation of Schlemm's canal with the OMNI Surgical System. The black arrow marks the tip of the device's cannula. Through the blue microcatheter, viscodilation of Schlemm's canal (brownish shading) is clearly visible chronologically (A–F).

2.2 Canaloplasty + trabeculotomy

To perform the trabeculotomy, the same catheter is advanced once again through 180° of Schlemm's canal and withdrawn using a cheese-wire technique to unroof the canal.

2.3 Canaloplasty (+ trabeculotomy) + cataract surgery

In ab-interno canaloplasty combined with cataract surgery, the surgical steps are almost unchanged. Only the microincision of 2.2 mm is slightly larger and access to the anterior chamber with the OMNI Surgical System is via the cataract incision.

3. OMNI Surgical System: scientific status

The first single-incision approaches to trabeculectomy for glaucoma treatment only allowed trabeculectomy over 120° [21, 22]. A further development of this approach allowed trabeculectomy over a full 360° range. In the new approach, entry and exit from Schlemm's canal is through a single incision. A blue coloration of the suture material used made it possible to control with a gonioscope the exact placement and the accurate penetration of Schlemm's canal with the suture material. The first application of this technique was developed for congenital glaucoma. Furthermore, better results were obtained in direct comparison with the 360° technique than with the 120° technique [23–25].

Canaloplasty is based on the finding that the IOP-lowering effect of canalostomy is more likely due to viscodilation of Schlemm's canal and the resulting disruption of the lateral walls, inner wall endothelium, and bridging structures. Thus, in contrast to trabeculotomy, canaloplasty targets not only the inner wall and trabecular meshwork but also distal outflow resistance [26].

Ab-interno canaloplasty differs from ab-externo canaloplasty in that Schlemm's canal is accessed through the anterior chamber via a small goniotomy, and therefore only a small clear corneal incision is required, rather than conjunctival dissection and scleral flap. There is no tensioning suture [22].

3.1 Ab-interno canaloplasty

To prevent the sometimes serious side effects of trabeculectomy, such as shallow anterior chamber, uncontrolled hypotony, choroidal detachment, and macular wrinkles, non-penetrating filtering techniques have been proposed.

Non-penetrating filtering surgery, such as canaloplasty, involves techniques that focus on widening the Schlemm's canal to facilitate aqueous humor outflow via the physiologic pathway. The aim is to remove mechanical obstructions in the collector channels by improving aqueous humor outflow and creating additional pathways. Viscodilation separates the trabecular lamellae and creates microperforations in the inner wall of Schlemm's canal, allowing improved diffusion of aqueous humor through the proximal system into the distal system [4, 27].

The goal of this ab-interno canaloplasty is to restore physiologic aqueous humor outflow pathways independent of external wound healing. Numerous studies have demonstrated that canaloplasty is a relatively safe and effective surgical procedure that lowers intraocular pressure with continued pressure control over several years.

Additionally, postoperative management is simpler and fewer complications occur than with trabeculectomy [28–30].

In 2022, Toneatto et al. published retrospective interim results on ab-internal viscodilation of Schlemm's canal with the OMNI Surgical System in primary open-angle glaucoma (POAG) [4]. The primary endpoint at 12-month follow-up was defined as the proportion of eyes achieving an intraocular pressure of 18 mmHg or below, with an IOP reduction of more than 25% from baseline, either with the same number or fewer IOP-lowering medications and without additional IOP-lowering surgery or laser. In their cohort, the mean IOP reduction at 12 months compared to baseline was of 26.8% (from 23.0 ± 5.7 mmHg to 15.6 ± 3.6 mmHg). The mean number of medications at 12 months decreased from 3.0 ± 1.1 to 2.0 ± 1.4. Further publications reported comparable results [17, 31–33]. The results showed that surgery resulted in effective control and reduction of intraocular pressure. Only a few adverse events have occurred. Due to physiological blood regurgitation from Schlemm's canal, microhyphema was frequently observed; however, these microhyphema were not considered adverse events. 2 of 73 eyes showed clinically significant hyphema with more than 1 mm. In these two eyes, anterior chamber irrigation was performed without further postoperative complications affecting vision. Hyphema rates reported in the literature for ab-internal canaloplasties range from 0 to 20%, with the higher rates based mostly on studies that included milder hyphema. Mild postoperative hypotony (4–5 mmHg) occurred in 4 of 73 eyes within the first month but resolved without any intervention. No shallow anterior chambers or choroidal detachments were noted. IOP fluctuated widely during the first 30 days after surgery because antiglaucoma drops were discontinued after surgery and steroids were administered during the first weeks.

3.2 Ab-interno canaloplasty and trabeculectomy

In 2021 Klabe et al. [17] published a retrospective analysis of data drawn from existing health records. Prior surgery, patients were washed out of their ocular hypertensive medications according to generally accepted wash-out periods for prostaglandin analogs, beta blockers, alpha antagonists, and carbonic anhydrase inhibitors. All operations were performed by the same surgeon. In the sample of 38 eyes of 27 patients with open-angle glaucoma undergoing trabeculotomy/viscodilation using the OMNI Surgical System. 28 eyes were pseudophakic. 12- and 24-month results revealed statistically significant and clinically relevant reductions in intraocular pressure and medications. IOP decreased from 24.6 ± 3.0 mmHg to 14.7 ± 1.6 mmHg (40% IOP reduction from baseline) and 14.9 ± 2.0 mmHg (39%), respectively. Number of medications decreased from 1.9 ± 0.7 to 0.4 ± 0.6 and 0.5 ± 0.7, respectively. All retrospectively examined eyes showed a reduction in intraocular pressure of more than 20% from baseline. In addition, 83 and 85% of eyes required less medication than before MIGS treatment, and 63 and 58% of eyes were even medication-free. These outcomes were achieved without significant adverse events.

Another retrospective observation with a 12-month outcome was the ROMEO study [32]. This was a multicenter, retrospective, observational, single-arm study to evaluate the safety and effectiveness of canaloplasty and trabeculotomy with the OMNI Surgical System in pseudophakic eyes with OAG. Eyes were stratified by baseline IOP, with group 1 > 18 mmHg and group 2 ≤ 18 mmHg. Each group included 24 eyes of 24 patients. Surgeries were performed in 10 multi-subspecialty ophthalmic practices. Primary success was defined as the proportion of patients with at least 20% reduction in IOP from baseline or an IOP between 6 and 18 mmHg and on the same or fewer medications without secondary surgical intervention up to 12 months after MIGS. Mean IOP was reduced in group 1 from 21.8 ± 3.3 mmHg to 15.6 ± 2.4 mmHg (28%) and in group 2 from 15.4 ± 2.0 mmHg to 13.9 ± 3.5 mmHg (10%). Medications went from 1.7 ± 1.3 to 1.2 ± 1.3 and from 2.0 ± 1.3 to 1.3 ± 1.3, respectively. 91 and 90% of eyes, respectively, required less medication than before MIGS treatment.

Further results of retrospective observations after trabeculotomy/viscodilation with the OMNI Surgical System are comparable and in the same range as results reported here [18, 33].

The observed reduction in intraocular pressure and medication are clinically relevant to glaucoma progression and patient adherence. In eyes with progressive open-angle glaucoma despite medication therapy, a 20% or greater reduction in intraocular pressure has been shown to significantly reduce the risk of further progression of glaucoma [34]. This is one reason why the FDA accepts a 20% reduction in intraocular pressure as an endpoint in MIGS registry studies [35]. Reducing medication offers patients several benefits such as: increased treatment adherence, reduced exposure to topical glaucoma medications, slower progression of dry eye symptoms, and also time and money savings.

3.3 Ab-interno canaloplasty/trabeculectomy standalone or combined with cataract surgery

Previous studies have shown that cataract surgery (phacoemulsification) alone results in an average IOP reduction of 1.4 mmHg in glaucoma patients up to 3 years out from surgery [36]. To date, there have been no randomized clinical trials in which cataract surgery was performed with and without a MIGS with the OMNI Surgical System or in which cataract surgery was combined with the OMNI Surgical System device and then compared with cataract surgery combined with another MIGS procedure. Therefore, the effect of phacoemulsification on IOP lowering cannot be accurately determined or compared when the procedure is performed in combination with canaloplasty or canaloplasty/trabeculoplasty using the OMNI Surgical System.

A retrospective, consecutive case series from a single center reported a smaller but statistically non-significant reduction in intraocular pressure and medication use after combined surgery compared with MIGS surgery alone [31]. A total of 89 eyes were examined, the surgery was performed as standalone with OMNI Surgical System in 17 eyes and in 72 eyes in combination with a phacoemulsification. After 18 months, 5 and 17 eyes could still be analyzed, respectively. The observation was not randomized, therefore the influence of confounding variables cannot be ruled out. In addition, the small sample size may not have been powered adequately to show any difference. This study is also limited by the weaknesses inherent to retrospective studies including selection bias and variable follow-up.

The second part of the ROMEO study (see Section 3.2 above) provides 12-month results after combined surgery of canaloplasty/trabeculotomy with the OMNI Surgical System and cataract surgery in patients with mild to moderate OAG [37]. Group 1 included 24 eyes and group 2 included 57 eyes. Surgeries were performed in 11 multi-subspecialty ophthalmic practices. Mean IOP was reduced in group 1 from 21.9 ± 3.7 mmHg to 15.1 ± 3.7 mmHg (31%) and in group 2 from 14.1 ± 2.5 mmHg to 13.4 ± 3.1 mmHg (7%). Medications went from 2.0 ± 1.3 to 1.1 ± 1.1 and from 1.6 ± 1.3 to 0.9 ± 1.2, respectively. 88% and 91% of eyes, respectively, required the same or less medication than before MIGS treatment. No safety issues were identified based on the analysis of adverse events and visual acuity.

The GEMINI clinical trial evaluated the efficacy of combined canaloplasty/trabeculotomy surgery with the OMNI Surgical System and cataract surgery in patients with mild to moderate glaucoma. 113 eyes with POAG were treated in 15 multi-subspecialty ophthalmic practices. Mean unmedicated diurnal IOP was reduced from 23.9 ± 3.0 mmHg at baseline to 15.4 ± 3.8 mmHg (36%) at month 12. Medications went from 1.8 ± 0.9 to 0.3 ± 0.9. 78% of eyes required less medication than before MIGS treatment.

Nevertheless, these and similar results [4] show that there are no significant disadvantages for the glaucoma patient when the OMNI Surgical System is combined with phacoemulsification. Rather, the advantage for both patient and physician is the ability to treat both cataract and aqueous humor outflow with only one surgical procedure, just one scleral incision.

3.4 Other glaucoma than primary open-angle glaucoma

There is limited data available on the performance of OMNI Surgical System in pseudoexfoliation glaucoma and pigmentary glaucoma [5]. One retrospective observation included only six patients diagnosed with pseudoexfoliation and one with pigmentary glaucoma [32] and another clinical study includes nine and one patients, respectively [20]. In general, the demographics of these patients were unremarkable compared with the pooled study populations. No clinically significant differences were observed compared to the results from patients with primary open-angle glaucoma. This observed effect suggests that OMNI Surgical System is also effective in secondary open angel glaucoma. However, the number of patients in these two studies is too small to draw any conclusions about the relative efficacy of the OMNI Surgical System for treating these types of glaucoma.

Although OMNI Surgical System is primarily used for open-angle glaucoma in adults, the combination of ab-interno canaloplasty and trabeculotomy is also useful for childhood glaucoma. Ab-interno trabeculotomy is the treatment of choice for primary congenital and other pediatric glaucoma. A retrospective study evaluated the results of a group of 46 eyes with various pediatric glaucoma treated with TRAB360, a precursor to OMNI Surgical System without canaloplasty function. Success was achieved in 81% of eyes with primary congenital glaucoma [38].

3.5 Combined MIGS

To date, few data are available on the combined use of the OMNI Surgical System with another MIGS technique. At the 2022 Annual Meeting of the American Society of Cataract and Refractive Surgery, a case series of 16 glaucomatous eyes undergoing combined surgery with the Hydrus Microstent (Ivantis, Irvine, CA, USA) and a canaloplasty with OMNI Surgical System was presented for the first time. In 2022 [39], there was another case report of 8 eyes in which the two devices were used during one glaucoma surgery [40]. In both case series, a significant and clinically meaningful reduction in IOP occurred in the majority of patients. Only in some patients in the case series could the number of IOP-lowering agents be reduced to achieve the target IOP. In patients with uncontrolled IOP who are already receiving maximally tolerated medication therapy, implantation of a hydrus microstent alone with OMNI Surgical System canaloplasty may not be an effective means of reducing medication burden.

Nevertheless, it can be concluded from these case series that a combination of ab-interno canaloplasty with the OMNI Surgical System with another MIGS technique is still a relatively safe and well tolerated method to control intraocular pressure. And in patients who have not achieved an adequate response of intraocular pressure despite the combined procedure, it is important to know that this does not preclude or prevent further glaucoma surgeries.

3.6 Clinical trials

The OMNI Surgical System has only been on the market for a few years. Therefore, only a few clinical studies are currently listed on the official website of the U.S. National Library of Medicine (ClinicalTrials.gov). By February 2023, 3, studies will be or have been conducted in the USA (NCT04530084, NCT03861169, NCT04872348) and one study in Poland (NCT04503356). No clinical trial is registered on the European website (clinicaltrialsregister.eu). All other peer-reviewed publications published to date are retrospective observations or case reports from single or multiple sites.

The first final 12-month analysis of a clinical trial was published in 2022 [20]. The GEMINI study was a prospective, multicenter, interventional, single-arm clinical study of patients with mild-moderate OAG undergoing 360° canaloplasty followed by 180° trabeculotomy with the OMNI Surgical System at the time of phacoemulsification. Final results from the 120 eyes analyzed showed that both IOP and the need for IOP-lowering medications were significantly reduced for at least 12 months postoperatively, with an excellent safety profile and no serious adverse event. Mean diurnal IOP without medication was reduced by 34%, with 84% of eyes having IOP reduced by more than 20% from baseline. Mean medication use was reduced by 78%, and 80% were medication-free at month 12. In this study, there was no control group, so the IOP-lowering effect of phacoemulsification alone or the effect of OMNI Surgical System compared with other MIGS could not be comparatively investigated.

3.7 Limitations

The current status of the clinical observations reported in this chapter is limited by some of the following factors:

Most are retrospective, uncontrolled studies with few or only one site (sometimes only one surgeon). Most are non-comparative, non-hypothesis-testing, descriptive studies with an inhomogeneous patient selection. Therefore, the occurring effects in terms of IOP and number of glaucoma medications are underestimated rather than overestimated compared to a prospective study with precisely defined inclusion and exclusion criteria.

Glaucoma is a chronic disease. In contrast, the longest observation period to date after MIGS with the OMNI Surgical System of 24 months is a relatively short period. However, this time frame is long enough to capture intraoperative and postoperative safety events as well as early surgical failures.

Completely standardized methods for ophthalmic measurements, surgical interventions, and medication initiation or discontinuation are the norm in a prospective study but not possible in a retrospective study. The decision to washout and to decrease or increase a patient's medication was made solely within the context of a surgeon's medical practice.

Some eyes had previously undergone other glaucoma surgery, such as trabeculectomy, deep sclerectomy, or also other MIGS. These patients were included based on the results of previous studies showing that canaloplasty can be successfully performed even in patients with failed trabeculectomy in whom Schlemm's canal remained largely undamaged by previous filtering surgery [41, 42].

4. Conclusion

MIGS are considered for patients with mild to moderate visual field defects when medication therapy does not result in sufficient pressure reduction or IOP is above target pressure, patients do not adhere to therapy, or patients are suspected of not adhering to therapy, resulting in an increased risk of glaucoma progression. Especially, by reducing the number of different topical medications, MIGS are a useful tool to improve patient adherence and thus treatment outcomes. In addition, earlier intervention may help delay or avoid the need for more invasive surgery.

The OMNI Surgical System provides a practical approach to treating conventional outflow resistance by sequential canaloplasty and trabeculotomy, proximal to the juxtacanalicular trabecular meshwork and the inner wall of Schlemm's canal, and distal to Schlemm's canal and collecting channels.

Canaloplasty and trabeculotomy with the OMNI Surgical System as a standalone procedure or in combination with cataract surgery results in clinically relevant and statistically significant reductions in both IOP and IOP medication with an excellent safety profile. The procedure should be considered for eyes with mild to moderate open-angle glaucoma that require a safe and effective surgical intervention to achieve a reduction in intraocular pressure, a reduction in medication, or both. Phakic eyes can be treated as well as pseudophakic eyes.

Acknowledgements

Dr. Karsten Klabe reports grants from Sight Sciences, Inc., manufacturer of the OMNI Surgical System. Dr. Andreas Fricke has nothing to disclose.

Conflict of interest

The authors declare no conflict of interest.

Author details

Karsten Klabe* and Andreas Fricke
Internationale Innovative Ophthalmochirurgie, Düsseldorf, Germany

*Address all correspondence to: studien.k.klabe@augenchirurgie.clinic

References

[1] European Glaucoma Society. Terminology and Guidelines for Glaucoma. 5th ed. Savona, Italy: PubliComm; 2021

[2] Lavia C, Dallorto L, Maule M, Ceccarelli M, Fea AM. Minimally-invasive glaucoma surgeries (MIGS) for open angle glaucoma: A systematic review and meta-analysis. PLoS One. 2017;**12**(8):e0183142

[3] Brusini P, Filacorda S. Enhanced Glaucoma Staging System (GSS 2) for classifying functional damage in glaucoma. Journal of Glaucoma. 2006;**15**(1):40-46

[4] Toneatto G, Zeppieri M, Papa V, Rizzi L, Salati C, Gabai A, et al. 360° ab-interno schlemm's canal viscodilation with OMNI viscosurgical systems for open-angle glaucoma-midterm results. Journal of Clinical Medicine. 2022;**11**(1):259

[5] Dickerson JE, Dhamdhere K. Combined circumferential canaloplasty and trabeculotomy ab Interno with the OMNI surgical system. Frontiers in Ophthalmology. 2021;**1**(2):1-9

[6] Nordstrom BL, Friedman DS, Mozaffari E, Quigley HA, Walker AM. Persistence and adherence with topical glaucoma therapy. American Journal of Ophthalmology. 2005;**140**(4):598-606

[7] Hoffmann EM, Hengerer F, Klabe K, Schargus M, Thieme H, Voykov B. Glaucoma surgery today. Der Ophthalmologe. 2021;**118**(3):239-247

[8] Higginbotham EJ, Hansen J, Davis EJ, Walt JG, Guckian A. Glaucoma medication persistence with a fixed combination versus multiple bottles. Current Medical Research and Opinion. 2009;**25**(10):2543-2547

[9] Sleath B, Blalock SJ, Covert D, Skinner AC, Muir KW, Robin AL. Patient race, reported problems in using glaucoma medications, and adherence. ISRN Ophthalmology. 2012;**2012**:902819

[10] Tapply I, Broadway DC. Improving adherence to topical medication in patients with glaucoma. Patient Preference and Adherence. 2021;**15**:1477-1489

[11] Zaharia AC, Dumitrescu OM, Radu M, Rogoz RE. Adherence to therapy in glaucoma treatment—A review. Journal of Personalized Medicine. 2022;**12**(4):514

[12] Heijl A, Alm A, Bengtsson B, Bergström A, Calissendorff B, Lindblom B, et al. The glaucoma guidelines of the Swedish ophthalmological society. Acta Ophthalmologica. Supplement. 2012;**251**:1-40

[13] Saheb H, Ahmed IIK. Micro-invasive glaucoma surgery: Current perspectives and future directions. Current Opinion in Ophthalmology. 2012;**23**(2):96-104

[14] Wang J, Barton K. In: Sng CCA, Barton K, editors. Minimally Invasive Glaucoma Surgery [Internet]. Singapore: Springer; 2021. Available from: http://link.springer.com/10.1007/978-981-15-5632-6

[15] Terveen DC, Sarkisian SR, Vold SD, Selvadurai D, Williamson BK, Ristvedt DG, et al. Canaloplasty and trabeculotomy with the OMNI® surgical system in OAG with prior trabecular

microbypass stenting. International Ophthalmology. 2022 [Online ahead of print]

[16] Francis BA, Akil H, Bert BB. Ab interno Schlemm's canal surgery. Developments in Ophthalmology. 2017;**59**:127-146

[17] Klabe K, Kaymak H. Standalone trabeculotomy and viscodilation of Schlemm's canal and collector channels in open-angle glaucoma using the OMNI surgical system: 24-month outcomes. Clinical Ophthalmology. 2021;**15**:3121-3129

[18] Ondrejka S, Körber N, Dhamdhere K. Long-term effect of canaloplasty on intraocular pressure and use of intraocular pressure-lowering medications in patients with open-angle glaucoma. Journal of Cataract and Refractive Surgery. 2022;**48**(12):1388-1393

[19] Porsia L, Nicoletti M. Combined viscodilation of Schlemm's canal and collector channels and 360° ab-Interno trabeculotomy for congenital glaucoma associated with sturge-weber syndrome. International Medical Case Reports Journal. 2020;**13**:217-220

[20] Gallardo MJ, Pyfer MF, Vold SD, Sarkisian SR, Campbell A, Singh IP, et al. Canaloplasty and trabeculotomy combined with phacoemulsification for glaucoma: 12-month results of the GEMINI study. Clinical Ophthalmology. 2022;**16**:1225-1234

[21] Smith R. A new technique for opening the canal of Schlemm. Preliminary report. British Journal of Ophthalmology. 1960;**44**(6):370-373

[22] Dickerson JE, Brown RH. Circumferential canal surgery: A brief history. Current Opinion in Ophthalmology. 2020;**31**(2):139-146

[23] Beck AD, Lynch MG. 360 degrees trabeculotomy for primary congenital glaucoma. Archives of Ophthalmology. 1995;**113**(9):1200-1202

[24] Girkin CA, Rhodes L, McGwin G, Marchase N, Cogen MS. Goniotomy versus circumferential trabeculotomy with an illuminated microcatheter in congenital glaucoma. Journal of AAPOS. 2012;**16**(5):424-427

[25] Lim ME, Neely DE, Wang J, Haider KM, Smith HA, Plager DA. Comparison of 360-degree versus traditional trabeculotomy in pediatric glaucoma. Journal of AAPOS. 2015;**19**(2):145-149

[26] Smit BA, Johnstone MA. Effects of viscoelastic injection into Schlemm's canal in primate and human eyes: Potential relevance to viscocanalostomy. Ophthalmology. 2002;**109**(4):786-792

[27] Grieshaber MC, Pienaar A, Olivier J, Stegmann R. Comparing two tensioning suture sizes for 360 degrees viscocanalostomy (canaloplasty): A randomised controlled trial. Eye (London, England). Singapore: Springer; 2010;**24**(7):1220-1226

[28] Lewis RA, von Wolff K, Tetz M, Koerber N, Kearney JR, Shingleton BJ, et al. Canaloplasty: Three-year results of circumferential viscodilation and tensioning of Schlemm canal using a microcatheter to treat open-angle glaucoma. Journal of Cataract and Refractive Surgery. 2011;**37**(4):682-690

[29] Bull H, von Wolff K, Körber N, Tetz M. Three-year canaloplasty outcomes for the treatment of open-angle glaucoma: European study

results. Graefe's Archive for Clinical and Experimental Ophthalmology. 2011;**249**(10):1537-1545

[30] Kerr NM, Wang J, Barton K. Minimally invasive glaucoma surgery as primary stand-alone surgery for glaucoma. Clinical & Experimental Ophthalmology. 2017;**45**(4):393-400

[31] Hughes T, Traynor M. Clinical results of ab interno canaloplasty in patients with open-angle glaucoma. Clinical Ophthalmology. 2020;**14**:3641-3650

[32] Vold SD, Williamson BK, Hirsch L, Aminlari AE, Cho AS, Nelson C, et al. Canaloplasty and trabeculotomy with the OMNI system in pseudophakic patients with open-angle glaucoma: The ROMEO study. Ophthalmology Glaucoma. 2021;**4**(2):173-181

[33] Grabska-Liberek I, Duda P, Rogowska M, Majszyk-Ionescu J, Skowyra A, Koziorowska A, et al. 12-month interim results of a prospective study of patients with mild to moderate open-angle glaucoma undergoing combined viscodilation of Schlemm's canal and collector channels and 360° trabeculotomy as a standalone procedure or combined with cataract surgery. European Journal of Ophthalmology. 2022;**32**(1):309-315

[34] Chauhan BC, Mikelberg FS, Artes PH, Balazsi AG, LeBlanc RP, Lesk MR, et al. Canadian glaucoma study: 3. Impact of risk factors and intraocular pressure reduction on the rates of visual field change. Archives of Ophthalmology. 2010;**128**(10):1249-1255

[35] U.S. Department of Health and Human Services. Premarket Studies of Implantable Minimally Invasive Glaucoma Surgical (MIGS) Devices Guidance for Industry and Food and Drug Administration Staff [Internet]. Available from: https://www.fda.gov/

[36] Shingleton BJ, Pasternack JJ, Hung JW, O'Donoghue MW. Three and five year changes in intraocular pressures after clear corneal phacoemulsification in open angle glaucoma patients, glaucoma suspects, and normal patients. Journal of Glaucoma. 2006;**15**(6):494-498

[37] Hirsch L, Cotliar J, Vold S, Selvadurai D, Campbell A, Ferreira G, et al. Canaloplasty and trabeculotomy ab interno with the OMNI system combined with cataract surgery in open-angle glaucoma: 12-month outcomes from the ROMEO study. Journal of Cataract and Refractive Surgery. 2021;**47**(7):907-915

[38] Areaux RG, Grajewski AL, Balasubramaniam S, Brandt JD, Jun A, Edmunds B, et al. Trabeculotomy ab Interno with the Trab360 device for childhood glaucomas. American Journal of Ophthalmology. 2020;**209**:178-186

[39] Wallace RT, Chaya C, Swiston C. Ab interno canaloplasty in combination with hydrus microstent for the treatment of glaucoma: A retrospective chart review. In: ASCRS Annual Meeting 2022: Session: SPS-217 Minimally Invasive GlaucomaSurgery (MIGS) III, Washington, DC. Singapore: Springer; 2022

[40] Creagmile J, Kim WI, Scouarnec C. Hydrus microstent implantation with OMNI surgical system ab interno canaloplasty for the management of open-angle glaucoma in phakic patients refractory to medical therapy. American Journal of Ophthalmology Case Reports. 2023;**29**:101749

[41] Brusini P, Tosoni C. Canaloplasty after failed trabeculectomy: A possible option. Journal of Glaucoma. 2014;**23**(1):33-34

[42] Wang H, Xin C, Han Y, Shi Y, Ziaei S, Wang N. Intermediate outcomes of ab externo circumferential trabeculotomy and canaloplasty in POAG patients with prior incisional glaucoma surgery. BMC Ophthalmology. 2020;**20**(1):389

Section 3

Cataract and Refractive Surgery

Chapter 4

Cataract Surgery in Microphthalmic Eyes

Tianyu Zheng, Yi Lu, Peimin Lin, Jie Xu and Ao Miao

Abstract

Microphthalmos is a congenital ocular abnormality that mainly manifests as a significant reduction in the size of the eye and is often associated with cataracts and other eye diseases. Due to its special anatomical features, cataract surgery in microphthalmos has a higher risk of intraoperative and postoperative complications and impaired visual prognosis and is associated with reduced intraocular lens (IOL) calculation accuracy. This chapter describes the characteristics of microphthalmic cataract surgery, the incidence of complications, classic and additional surgical procedures (e.g., phacoemulsification combined with prophylactic anterior lamellar sclerostomy, laser peripheral iridotomy, anterior segment vitrectomy, piggyback IOLs), and selection of IOL calculation formula.

Keywords: microphthalmos, nanophthalmos, cataract surgery, complications, prevention

1. Introduction

Microphthalmos is a congenital ocular dysplasia characterized by a small eye volume with or without dysplastic ocular structures. It has been reported that there are one to three patients with microphthalmia in every 10,000 newborns [1]. The relevant ocular malformations including cataract congenital corneal opacity chorioretinal coloboma retinal dysplasia and so on can cause visual impairment to various degrees and lead to amblyopia and even blindness [1]. Common complications of microphthalmos are congenital cataracts in adolescents and age-related cataracts in seniors. In general cataract surgery for patients with microphthalmos is challenging with poor prognosis due not only to abnormal ocular development but also to the great extent of surgical difficulty and complication rate. Possible complications such as uveal effusion or suprachoroidal hemorrhage glaucoma and corneal decompensation may seriously harm the visual outcomes by resulting in exudative retinal detachment optic nerve impairment and corneal opacity. In 1982 Singh et al. first reported cataract surgery in six patients with microphthalmia and concluded that intraocular surgery in microphthalmos can have disastrous consequences [2]. With gradual maturation of phacoemulsification (PE) and other additional surgical procedures the safety and effectiveness of cataract surgery for microphthalmos have improved [3, 4]. This chapter mainly describes the surgical effects of cataract surgery for microphthalmos different additional surgical procedures methods for preventing surgical complications and selection of intraocular lens (IOL) formulas.

2. Clinical features and diagnosis of microphthalmos

Microphthalmos is divided into three clinical subtypes based on the axial length (AL) and the anterior chamber depth (ACD) [5, 6]. (i) Small eye with a proportionally decreasing volume is characterized by short ACD and short AL and can be further divided into (a) simple microphthalmos or nanophthalmos with a normal morphology structure, and (b) complex microphthalmos associated with other congenital ocular anomalies. The diagnostic criterion is generally defined as AL < 20–21 mm, which is less than two standard deviations of the average AL of healthy people [7–10]. Wu et al. suggest that increased retinal-choroidal-scleral thickening (greater than 1.7 mm) should also be considered when diagnosing microphthalmos because the increased retinal-choroidal-scleral thickness can account for potential risks of glaucoma, uveal effusion, and other complications in microphthalmos [11]. (ii) A normal AL eye with a disproportionately narrow anterior segment is called relative anterior microphthalmos (RAM). The diagnostic criteria are corneal diameter (CD) <11 mm and ACD <2.2 mm [12]. (ii) Short AL eye with a normal anterior segment is diagnosed as axial high hyperopia eye characterized by normal ACD and short AL.

3. Cataract surgeries in microphthalmos

Cataracts are a common complication in microphthalmos. For instance, complex microphthalmos is often associated with congenital cataracts, and simple microphthalmos with age-related cataracts can occur in senior patients. Current surgical treatments for cataracts include extracapsular cataract extraction (ECCE), small-incision cataract surgery (SICS), and PE. Regarding which approach is the best choice for patients with microphthalmos, it is generally currently believed that PE is much safer. However, some studies have noted that the lower complication rate and better prognosis of PE are due to earlier surgical intervention [4, 7, 9, 10, 13]. Kohli et al. suggested that surgical procedures should be selected according to the patient's biometric measurements and the cataract severity. For patients with microphthalmia, PE is recommended for soft cataracts in eyes with CD >8 mm and SICS for hard cataracts in eyes with CD ranging between 6 mm and 8 mm [13]. In conclusion, as long as the CD and rigidity of cataract nuclei permit, PE is considered the preferred surgical procedure for cataracts in microphthalmos.

Treatment for cataracts in microphthalmos has been a major challenge in ophthalmic surgery. The unsatisfactory prognosis is due not only to abnormal ocular development but also to the narrowed operating space. A shallow anterior chamber and small cornea can lead to more difficult operative procedures and a higher incidence of complications. In 1982, Singh et al. first reported cataract extraction in six microphthalmic eyes, with disastrous outcomes [2]. However, with the gradual development of PE and other surgical techniques, the safety and effectiveness of microphthalmic cataract surgery have improved significantly [3, 4]. Multiple studies have found that the current routine surgery, namely, PE combined with intraocular lens (IOL) implantation, achieves satisfactory therapeutic effects in patients with microphthalmia and cataracts [9, 14–16]. However, including patients with relatively long AL (inclusion criteria: AL < 20.0–21.0 mm) in these studies may be the actual reason for the good surgical outcomes, as shorter AL is a significant risk factor for surgical complications [9, 14–16]. It has been reported that the total complication rate of cataract surgery is 15 times higher in eyes with AL < 20.00 mm than in those with AL < 20.00 ~ 20.99 mm [8, 9].

The author of this chapter investigated outcomes of cataract surgery in patients with extreme microphthalmos (eyes with extremely short AL or extremely small CD) [6], including microphthalmia patients with AL < 18 mm and CD < 8 mm and found that the outcome of routine PE alone was not ideal. The median best-corrected visual acuity (BCVA) score merely increased from preoperative baseline at 20/800 (equal to 0.025 in decimal visual acuity) to 20/160 (equal to 0.125 in decimal visual acuity) postoperatively. Indeed, 75% of patients still had low vision, with visual acuity lower than 20/60 (equal to 0.3 in decimal visual acuity), and 25% remained blind, with only postoperative hand motion (HM). In particular, the vision of patients with complex microphthalmia did not improve at all. The high incidence of complications is an important reason for the poor postoperative outcome of cataract surgery in extreme microphthalmos. The incidence of severe complications reaches 16.7%, much higher than that in normal eye cataract surgery ("severe complications" include uveal effusion syndrome (UES), suprachoroidal hemorrhage (SCH), retinal detachment, corneal endothelial decompensation, intraoperative posterior capsule rupture, etc.). Therefore, lowering the rate of complications in extreme microphthalmic cataract surgery is an urgent goal.

4. Prevention of complications in microphthalmos cataract surgery

With modern cataract surgical techniques, microphthalmic eyes are no longer a restriction for cataract surgery. Nonetheless, intraocular surgery in microphthalmos involves a complication rate of nearly 40–60% [17]. Common complications include UES (incidence rate: 2.63–15.79%) [7, 10, 16, 18, 19], SCH (incidence rate: 3.33–12.50%) [3, 4, 6, 11], glaucoma (incidence rate: 10.64–40.91%) [6, 20–23], and corneal endothelial edema (incidence rate: 0.87–75%) [6, 7, 18, 22, 24], among others. In general, appropriate additional surgical procedures can help prevent the occurrence of complications.

4.1 UES and SCH

UES and SCH are among the most severe complications of cataract surgery for microphthalmos and may lead to permanent vision impairment. UES is characterized by a series of fundus changes, such as subchoroidal fluid accumulation and exudative retinal detachment. The primary mechanism is congestion of choroidal veins due to compression of the vortex vein via a thickened sclera or a sudden drop in intraocular pressure (IOP) during surgery [25]. Moreover, UES may occur in unoperated eyes as well as during or after cataract surgery. Postoperative UES may also result from latent uveal effusion that existed before surgery [26]. With the development of modern surgical techniques, the incidence of UES has decreased owing to less intraoperative IOP fluctuation (incidence rate: 2.63–15.79%) [7, 10, 16, 18, 19]. Day et al. retrospectively analyzed outcomes of cataract surgery in 103 microphthalmic eyes, with only three eyes developing choroidal effusion (mean AL = 20.05 ± 1.55 mm, 14.60 –20.99 mm) [9]. Lu et al. performed PE and IOL implantation in 38 microphthalmic eyes, and only

1 eye developed exudative ciliochoroidal detachment (mean AL = 16.87 ± 1.02 mm, 15.32–18.49 mm) [19].

UES can progress to severe SCH, which often predicts poor visual prognosis. Specifically, choroidal effusion stretches the wall of ciliary arteries and leads to their rupture and bleeding into the suprachoroidal space. Influenced by the fluctuation in IOP, SCH may occur intraoperatively or postoperatively, with the latter being delayed SCH [27]. SCH can occur in all intraocular procedures, including cataract surgery, but is more commonly encountered in microphthalmos (incidence rate in microphthalmia patients: 3.33–12.50% [3, 4, 6, 11]; incidence rate in the healthy population: 0.03–0.06% [27]). In 2016, Lemos et al. reported that 1 of 14 nanophthalmic eyes (mean AL = 18.72 ± 2.23 mm, 14.00–20.45 mm) that underwent cataract surgery developed transient choroidal hemorrhage, recovering with a final BCVA of 0.15 logMAR [3]. In 2017, the author of this chapter reported cataract surgery in 30 microphthalmic eyes. In the simple microphthalmos group, SCH occurred in 1 of 11 eyes and resolved after two months, with the BCVA recovering from early postoperative HM to 20/100 (mean AL = 16.4 ± 0.8 mm) [6].

Some researchers recommend anterior lamellar sclerectomy and vortex vein decompression for UES prevention and treatment. These two procedures can create and maintain an outflow pathway for the fluid accumulated in the suprachoroidal cavity during or after surgery, and the latter can directly relieve compression of the thickened sclera on the vortex vein. Anterior lamellar sclerectomy refers to making a two-thirds thick scleral flap in size from 4 × 4 mm to 6 × 6 mm, 2–8 mm behind the limbus, with the posterior margin not beyond the equator of the eyeball. At the bottom of it, a "V"-shaped sclerotomy is generated, with the tip toward the limbus and 4 mm away from it; the length of each arm of the "V" is 1.5 mm. Additionally, the tip of the "V" (approximately 5 mm) is excised, and the sclerotomy is left open [28]. Wax et al. reported a 38-year-old female patient with bilateral nanophthalmos with acute angle-closure glaucoma (AL = 16 mm in both eyes) [28]. After pars plana vitrectomy combined with trabeculectomy, UES occurred in the left eye and disappeared after drainage by the anterior lamellar sclerectomy mentioned above. Prophylactic anterior lamellar sclerectomy was performed in her right eye before subsequent procedures. As a result, the IOP of the right eye was well controlled, and no UES occurred. Wang et al. reported a 29-year-old female patient with bilateral microphthalmos and angle-closure glaucoma (AL = 16.4 mm in both eyes). Her left eye developed UES after cataract extraction combined with trabeculectomy and peripheral iridectomy and recovered after anterior lamellar sclerectomy. In her right eye, prophylactic anterior lamellar sclerectomy followed by trabeculectomy, peripheral iridectomy, cataract extraction, and IOL implantation was performed. With stable postoperative IOP and the absence of UES in her right eye, this quadruple-combined operation had a credible preventive effect.

Vortex vein decompression refers to producing a rectangular scleral flap of 6 mm × 4 mm with long edges parallel to the equator at 4 mm in front of the outlet of the vortex vein. On this premise, the vortex vein is gradually separated backward, and a 2 mm × 2 mm deeper scleral incision is made in front of the vortex vein near the long edge of the scleral flap. Skipping the eyeball's 3 and 9 o'clock direction is vital to avoid injury to the long posterior ciliary artery and nerves [10, 29]. Recent clinical studies have confirmed the safety and effectiveness of vortex vein decompression in cataract surgery for microphthalmos. In 2017, Rajendrababu et al. conducted a randomized controlled trial to compare differences in surgical complications and visual outcomes between a sclerostomy group (cataract surgery combined with prophylactic vortex vein decompression) and control group (cataract surgery alone) (mean AL of the sclerostomy group = 17.50 ± 1.31 mm; mean AL of the control group = 18.71 ± 1.33 mm). Multivariate model analysis of 60 nanophthalmic eyes showed that prophylactic use of vortex vein decompression was associated with a lower risk of complications than cataract surgery alone (odds ratio: 0.20) but without a significant effect on the prognosis of vision and postoperative IOP [10]. In 2021, the same research team reported a retrospective study of cataract surgery in 114 nanophthalmic patients (mean AL = 17.64 ± 1.74 mm, 14.5 mm – 20.5 mm). The incidence of UES in the sclerostomy group (cataract surgery with prophylactic vortex vein decompression) was significantly lower than that in the control group (cataract surgery alone) (incidence rate of UES in sclerostomy group: 7.84%; incidence rate of UES in control group: 22.22%), though the difference in visual outcome between the two groups was not analyzed [7].

It should be noted that the scleral incision may result in new complications, including iatrogenic retinal tears, fibrovascular in-growth into the sclerostomy site, and vitreous incarceration [10, 30]. Hoffman et al. suggested that the combination of sclerectomy and cataract surgery should be considered cautiously. For existing UES, sclerostomy should be performed several weeks before cataract surgery. To prevent intraoperative and postoperative UES, prophylactic application of mannitol or acetazolamide 30 minutes before surgery to reduce vitreous volume may be a safer alternative to additional surgical procedures [31].

4.2 Glaucoma

Glaucoma is a comorbidity of microphthalmos and a common postoperative complication after cataract surgery. In microphthalmic eyes, the anatomical basis for angle-closure glaucoma is a short AL, short ACD, and narrowed anterior chamber angle. The lens is disproportionally larger and thicker compared with the volume of microphthalmos, and the area where the lens is close to the iris increases, leading to a higher risk of pupillary block. In microphthalmic eyes, angle-closure glaucoma is common before surgery, but both open-angle and angle-closure glaucoma after surgery have been reported [19, 32]. The onset of postoperative open-angle glaucoma is relatively late, usually several years after surgery and may not be directly related to the operation but to anterior segment dysplasia, including malformation of the trabecular meshwork and the Schlemm canal [23, 32].

Cataract extraction combined with IOL implantation can relieve lens-derived narrow anterior chamber angle conditions and achieve the therapeutic effect of deepening the anterior chamber. However, one study found that compared with normal eyes, patients with microphthalmos are more likely to have peripheral anterior synechiae (PAS) [19]. As a result, the postoperative effect of angle opening is often poor, and the IOP even increases slightly in microphthalmic eyes. Additionally, the success rate of combined goniosynechialysis with cataract surgery is low [19]. The author of this chapter found AL, ACD, and the degree of angle closure before surgery to be closely related to the likelihood of developing postoperative glaucoma [6]. In infants with microphthalmos, extremely early surgical intervention may be an important trigger of postoperative glaucoma [20, 21]. Praveen et al. suggested that to minimize the complication rate without compromising the final potential visual outcomes, cataract surgery in microphthalmic eyes should be postponed until the end of the first month of life [21].

Peripheral iridectomy (PI) is a common prophylactic surgical procedure used to prevent angle-closure glaucoma in microphthalmos. The dilemma between the crowded anterior segment and the normal-sized lens leads to an extremely narrowed aqueous passage on the iris's posterior surface and the lens's anterior surface, resulting in a high risk of pupillary block in microphthalmia patients. PI eliminates the pressure difference between the anterior and posterior chambers and is a standard treatment for correcting pupillary block. To date, the combination of PI and cataract surgery has achieved high recognition among ophthalmic specialists for treating microphthalmic cataracts. Prasad et al. applied PI, posterior capsulotomy, and anterior vitrectomy in combination with phacoaspiration in 37 microphthalmic infant eyes and indicated that prophylactic PI and adequate vitrectomy can reduce glaucoma incidence (mean AL = 15.76 ± 0.56 mm, 14.66–16.41 mm) [33]. Furthermore, Day and Seki et al. suggested that combined usage of PI and cataract surgery in patients at high risk of malignant glaucoma (microphthalmic eye with AL < 20 mm) may facilitate future laser zonulotomy or hyaloidotomy if aqueous misdirection occurs [9 34]. Nevertheless, Steijns et al. conducted retrospective analysis of 43 nanophthalmic eyes and found no significant correlation between PI and occurrence of postoperative angle-closure glaucoma. These authors believed that the decision to perform intraoperative PI should be based on the degree of angle closure and the individual risk of postoperative angle-closure glaucoma (average AL = 20.01 mm, 15.47–20.48 mm) [16]. The discrepant conclusions of the retrospective studies by Prasad and Steijns may be associated with differences in the mean AL of the included patients. The possibility that PI has a more significant anti-glaucoma effect in eyes with shorter ALs cannot be ruled out and needs to be verified.

Postoperative malignant glaucoma is one of the most serious complications of cataract surgery for microphthalmos. The pathogenesis involves backward flows of the aqueous humor, becoming trapped in the anterior vitreous cavity and resulting in an elevation in posterior segment pressure and a forward movement of the lens-iris diaphragm, which further obstruct the aqueous humor flow. Once a vicious cycle forms, the anterior chamber will become progressively shallow, and the IOP will increase continuously [35, 36]. Despite the development of surgical techniques, malignant glaucoma is still frequently reported after microphthalmic cataract surgery (incidence rate: 1.85–9.52%) [6, 9, 18, 19, 37, 38]. In 2013, Day et al. reported seven cases of malignant glaucoma among 103 postcataract surgery microphthalmic eyes (mean AL = 20.05 ± 1.55, 14.60–20.99 mm) [9]. In 2015, Ye et al. reported two cases of malignant glaucoma among 89 nanophthalmic eyes after cataract surgery (mean AL = 19.24 ± 1.20 mm, 15.82–20.97 mm) [18], and Rajendrababu et al. diagnosed one case of secondary malignant glaucoma after cataract surgery among 19 nanophthalmic eyes (mean AL = 18.6 ± 1.8 mm, 17.7–19.5 mm) in 2021 [39].

The principle for treating malignant glaucoma is to communicate the anterior chamber to the vitreous cavity to relieve obstruction at the interface between the ciliary body and vitreous body [40]. Iridazolulohyaloid vitrectomy (IZHV), which was first proposed by Lois in 2001 [41], has been proven to be a safe and effective technique. This procedure creates a direct aqueous humor channel between the anterior chamber and the vitreous cavity, with a lower recurrence rate than for other operations (such as laser posterior capsulotomy or anterior vitrectomy). It is an applicable procedure for surgeons specializing in cataract surgery and is a good choice for treating or preventing malignant glaucoma intraoperatively and postoperatively [42]. For example, Zarnowski et al. used IZHV to treat 10 patients with pseudophakic malignant glaucoma and achieved a cure rate of 100% (mean AL = 21.30 ± 1.06 mm, 20.15–22.31 mm) [43]. The author of this chapter has also adopted this procedure and successfully treated a case of malignant glaucoma in complex microphthalmos with congenital zonular abnormality [6]. In summary, combining IZHV and cataract surgery for microphthalmia patients with a high risk of malignant glaucoma may achieve an ideal outcome, but further investigation is needed.

4.3 Corneal edema and endothelial decompensation

An impaired corneal endothelium is an important factor affecting the visual prognosis of microphthalmia patients after cataract surgery. Corneal endothelial injury presents as corneal edema in the early stage, and in severe cases, it may gradually progress to corneal endothelial decompensation.

In intraocular surgery for microphthalmos, transient corneal edema is the most common early postoperative complication attributed to the reduced surgical space in a shallow anterior chamber and a small cornea. Both the proximity of the phaco probe to the cornea and the generation of excess heat energy result in mechanical and thermal damage to the corneal endothelium [39]. With the improvement in surgical technology, the incidence of corneal endothelial decompensation after microphthalmic cataract surgery has gradually decreased, despite high occurrence of corneal edema. Matalia et al. reported transient corneal edema in 22 of 47 eyes with microcornea after cataract surgery, with an incidence rate of 46.8% (mean CD = 8.6 ± 0.72 mm, 7–9.5 mm) [22]. Additionally, the author of this chapter reported that the incidence of postoperative transient corneal edema reaches 73% in all microphthalmia patients, with 100% in the RAM group (a total of 11 eyes, CD = 7.3 ± 1.0 mm, ACD = 1.15 ± 0.85 mm) [6]. However, except for two eyes in the RAM group that developed chronic corneal endothelial dysfunction, corneal edema in the other patients disappeared within one to two weeks.

Anterior vitrectomy combined with cataract surgery is an effective method to solve the problem of anterior segment narrowness in microphthalmic eyes. When combined with posterior capsulotomy, anterior vitrectomy can prevent visual axis opacification, the most common complication of pediatric cataract surgery, caused by anterior vitreous fibrosis and posterior capsular opacification [44]. Moreover, anterior vitrectomy helps to reduce the volume of the vitreous body and deepen the anterior chamber while decreasing the difficulty of cataract surgery and the risk of corneal endothelial injury in microphthalmic eyes [45]. Recently, phacoaspiration with primary posterior capsulotomy and anterior vitrectomy has achieved satisfactory results in clinical treatment for microphthalmos with congenital cataract [21, 33, 45]. Praveen et al. applied cataract surgery combined with anterior vitrectomy in 72 congenital cataract eyes with microphthalmos and found only four cases of visual axis opacification and no corneal edema (mean AL of the right eye: 16.7 ± 1.5 mm; mean AL of the left eye: 16.6 ± 1.3 mm) [21]. Prasad et al. combined PE, PI, primary posterior capsulotomy, and anterior vitrectomy in 37 microphthalmic eyes of 20 infants with congenital cataracts; only two eyes developed visual axis opacification, and no corneal edema occurred postoperatively (mean AL = 15.76 ± 0.56 mm, 14.66–16.41 mm) [33].

In regard to treatment of cataracts in adult microphthalmic eyes, clinicians should balance the benefits of anterior vitrectomy with its risks. Anterior vitrectomy for microphthalmos can easily lead to posterior capsule rupture during cutting and penetrating procedures because the lens/eye volume ratio is approximately 25%, much larger than the 4% in the healthy population [16]. Additionally, a risk of retinal impairment exists during anterior vitrectomy due to the close proximity between the limbus and ora serrata region in microphthalmos [16]. Therefore, for adult microphthalmic cataract surgery, an individualized clinical decision on whether to combine anterior vitrectomy needs concrete analysis, including ACD, intraoperative visibility, and surgical techniques.

5. IOL implantation and formula selection in microphthalmic cataract surgery

Microphthalmic eyes usually present high hyperopia, which requires high IOL power. For adults, IOL implantation is necessary if the ocular condition permits. Regardless, several studies have noted that primary IOL implantation should be considered cautiously for microphthalmic children with congenital cataracts [20, 33]. First, implantation of an adult-sized IOL into the small eyeball of an infant with microphthalmia requires more precise surgical technique than routine cataract surgery. Second, owing to the growth of an infant's eyes, the change in postoperative refraction is more significant than in adults. The correction achieved with frame glasses or contact lenses for the aphakic eye may be more accurate than that with IOL implantation. In addition, primary IOL implantation may increase the incidence of postoperative complications such as secondary glaucoma and retinal detachment [20, 33, 46]. A study by Praveen et al. showed that even without IOL implantation, early surgical intervention and adequate amblyopia training can improve the visual acuity of children with microphthalmos and congenital cataracts [21].

5.1 Formula selection in microphthalmos cataract surgery

A unified standard for the most appropriate formula for microphthalmos has yet to be determined. Among conventional IOL formulas, the Hoffer Q formula is recommended by the Royal School of Ophthalmologists as the preferred formula for short eyes (AL ≤ 22 mm) [47]. However, several large-scale clinical studies have found that the Haigis formula outperforms the Hoffer Q formula [48–51]. Over the last decades, new-generation IOL formulas have emerged, as follows: formulas involving artificial intelligence (Hill-Radial Basis Function, Ladas Super Formula AI, Pearl-DGS formula); formulas using a combination of theoretical optics, thin lens formulas, and big data techniques (Kane formula); and formulas based on theoretical optics with regression and ray-tracing components (Olsen formula, Okulix formula). Among new-generation formulas, the Kane formula has been demonstrated to be relatively suitable for microphthalmic eyes in a few studies [50, 52, 53]. However, the update of the IOL formula is not equivalent to replacement. Luo et al.'s meta-analysis of 1476 microphthalmos (AL ≤22 mm) in 14 studies showed that the accuracy of new-generation formulas, such as Barrett Universal II and Kane, were generally superior to conventional IOL formulas (including the Haigis, Hoffer Q, SRK/T formulas) [54]. Moreover, Shrivastava and associates performed a meta-analysis of 15 studies involving 2395 short eyes (AL ≤22 mm) and concluded that there is no significant difference between the Barrett Universal II formula, the Olsen formula, and conventional IOL formulas (including the Haigis, Hoffer Q, SRK/T formulas) [55]. The author of this chapter also compared the accuracy of six IOL formulas (including the Haigis, Hoffer Q, Holladay I, SRK/T, Barrett Universal II, and Hoffer QST formulas) in nanophthalmos and RAM patients. When using the IOL Master 500 for biometric measurement (omitting the parameter of the lens thickness), the Haigis formula was the most accurate among the six IOL calculation formulas for cataract patients with nanophthalmos (mean AL = 16.84 ± 1.36 mm, 15.25–19.82 mm), whereas the Barrett Universal II formula showed the highest accuracy in cataract patients with RAM (mean CD = 8.41 ± 0.92 mm, 7.00–9.50 mm) [56]. Certain limitations in the new-generation formulas have been found, including requirements for more biometric parameters and specific instruments than traditional formulas and restrictions in calculating the IOL power of short eyes by the scope of the database [56]. As a result, application of new-generation formulas in nanophthalmos and RAM eyes needs further investigation.

5.2 Piggyback IOL implantation

Microphthalmos with high hyperopia usually requires high-power IOLs (generally greater than 40 diopters), which is generally out of the normal range and inaccessible in clinical practice [57]. In 1993, Gayton implanted two IOLs in the same eye for the first time, pioneering the procedure of piggyback IOL implantation [58]. However, this technique remains controversial among clinicians. Proponents believed that the piggyback technique has the advantage of a higher correction power and a greater postoperative benefit than traditional single-piece IOL implantation [57, 59], and opponents have concerns about its intraoperative safety. Because of the crowded anterior chamber and the fragile zonula, it is a challenge for surgeons to implant two IOLs in the same microphthalmos, which will certainly prolong the operation time and amplify the risk of intraoperative complications [8, 9]. This author's previous study reported that during piggyback IOL implantation, a patient with microphthalmos developed SCH after the first IOL was inserted into the capsule [6]. Moreover, with this approach, the unique postoperative complication interlenticular opacification severely impairs postoperative visual acuity [57].

In summary, implantation of a customized single IOL is the safest choice for microphthalmic eyes. If a high-power IOL cannot be obtained, experienced surgeons may adopt piggyback IOL implantation, placing two pieces of IOLs in the capsular bag and the sulcus, respectively [31, 57]. During the operation, attention should be given to thoroughly cleaning the capsule to minimize excessive proliferation of lens epithelial cells and avoid occurrence of interlenticular opacification [57].

6. Conclusion

Cataract surgery in microphthalmos is no longer forbidden, and PE is the first choice of surgical treatment. In microphthalmic eyes with a relatively long AL, PE can generally achieve satisfactory surgical outcomes. However, extreme microphthalmic eyes (with extremely short AL) still have a high risk of complications. Additional application of anterior lamellar sclerectomy or vortex vein decompression may be a good option to prevent UES and SCH. PI may reduce the incidence of postoperative angle-closure glaucoma, and the IZHV procedure can effectively treat or prevent malignant glaucoma. Anterior vitrectomy may be used to deepen the anterior chamber and reduce corneal endothelial damage. However, it should be noted that additional surgical procedures may bring new risks of complications.

Author details

Tianyu Zheng[1,2,3,4*], Yi Lu[1,2,3,4], Peimin Lin[1,2,3,4], Jie Xu[1,2,3,4] and Ao Miao[1,2,3,4]

1 Department of Ophthalmology, Eye and ENT Hospital, Fudan University, Shanghai, China

2 Eye Institute, Eye and ENT Hospital, Fudan University, Shanghai, China

3 Key Laboratory of Myopia, Ministry of Health, Shanghai, China

4 Shanghai Key Laboratory of Visual Impairment and Restoration, Shanghai, China

*Address all correspondence to: susu0102@163.com

References

[1] Plaisancié J et al. Genetics of anophthalmia and microphthalmia. Part 1: Non-syndromic anophthalmia/microphthalmia. Human Genetics. 2019;**138**:799-830

[2] Singh OS, Simmons RJ, Brockhurst RJ, Trempe CL. Nanophthalmos: A perspective on identification and therapy. Ophthalmology (Rochester, Minn.). 1982;**89**:1006

[3] Lemos JA et al. Cataract surgery in patients with Nanophthalmos: Results and complications. European Journal of Ophthalmology. 2016;**26**:103-106

[4] Yuzbasioglu E, Artunay O, Agachan A, Bilen H. Phacoemulsification in patients with nanophthalmos. Canadian Journal of Ophthalmology. 2009;**44**:534-539

[5] Parrish RK, Donaldson K, MellemKairala MB, Simmons RJ. Nanophthalmos, relative anterior microphthalmos, and axial hyperopia. In: Steinert RF, editor. Cataract surgery. 3rd edition. Saunders, Readfield, ME; 2009. pp. 389-400

[6] Zheng T et al. Outcomes and prognostic factors of cataract surgery in adult extreme Microphthalmos with axial length <18 mm or corneal diameter <8 mm. American Journal of Ophthalmology. 2017;**184**:84-96

[7] Rajendrababu S, Shroff S, Uduman MS, Babu N. Clinical spectrum and treatment outcomes of patients with nanophthalmos. Eye. 2021;**35**:825-830

[8] Day AC, MacLaren RE, Bunce C, Stevens JD, Foster PJ. Reply: Cataract surgery and microphthalmic eyes. Journal of Cataract and Refractive Surgery. 2013;**39**:818-819

[9] Day AC, MacLaren RE, Bunce C, Stevens JD, Foster PJ. Outcomes of phacoemulsification and intraocular lens implantation in microphthalmos and nanophthalmos. Journal of Cataract and Refractive Surgery. 2013;**39**:87-96

[10] Rajendrababu S et al. A randomized controlled trial comparing outcomes of cataract surgery in Nanophthalmos with and without prophylactic Sclerostomy. American Journal of Ophthalmology. 2017;**183**:125-133

[11] Wu W et al. Cataract surgery in patients with nanophthalmos. Journal of Cataract and Refractive Surgery. 2004;**30**:584-590

[12] Carifi G. Cataract surgery in eyes with Nanophthalmos and relative anterior Microphthalmos. American Journal of Ophthalmology. 2012;**154**:1005

[13] Kohli G et al. Cataract surgery in eyes with associated coloboma: Predictors of outcome and safety of different surgical techniques. Indian Journal of Ophthalmology. 2021;**69**:937

[14] Jung KI, Yang JW, Lee YC, Kim S. Cataract surgery in eyes with Nanophthalmos and relative anterior Microphthalmos. American Journal of Ophthalmology. 2012;**153**:1161-1168

[15] Carifi G, Safa F, Aiello F, Baumann C, Maurino V. Cataract surgery in small adult eyes. The British Journal of Ophthalmology. 2014;**98**:1261-1265

[16] Steijns D, Bijlsma WR, Van der Lelij A. Cataract surgery in patients with Nanophthalmos. Ophthalmology. 2013;**120**:266-270

[17] Carricondo PC, Andrade T, Prasov L, Ayres BM, Moroi SE. Nanophthalmos: A review of the clinical Spectrum and genetics. Journal of Ophthalmology. 2018;**2018**:1-9

[18] Ye Z et al. Outcomes of coaxial micro-incision phacoemulsification in Nanophthalmic eyes: Report of retrospective case series. Eye Science. 2015;**30**:94-100

[19] Lu Q, He W, Lu Y, Zhu X. Morphological features of anterior segment: Factors influencing intraocular pressure after cataract surgery in nanophthalmos. Eye Vision. 2020;7:47

[20] Vasavada VA et al. Intraoperative performance and postoperative outcomes of cataract surgery in infant eyes with microphthalmos. Journal of Cataract and Refractive Surgery. 2009;**35**:519-528

[21] Praveen MR, Vasavada AR, Shah SK, Khamar MB, Trivedi RH. Long-term postoperative outcomes after bilateral congenital cataract surgery in eyes with microphthalmos. Journal of Cataract and Refractive Surgery. 2015;**41**:1910-1918

[22] Matalia J, Shirke S, Shetty KB, Matalia H. Surgical outcome of congenital cataract in eyes with microcornea. Journal of Pediatric Ophthalmology and Strabismus. 2018;**55**:30-36

[23] Nishina S, Noda E, Azuma N. Outcome of early surgery for bilateral congenital cataracts in eyes with microcornea. American Journal of Ophthalmology. 2007;**144**:276-280

[24] Nihalani BR, Jani UD, Vasavada AR, Auffarth GU. Cataract surgery in relative anterior Microphthalmos. Ophthalmology. 2005;**112**:1360-1367

[25] Uyama M et al. Uveal effusion syndrome: Clinical features, surgical treatment, histologic examination of the sclera, and pathophysiology. Ophthalmology. 2000;**107**:441-449

[26] Sakai H et al. Uveal effusion in primary angle-closure glaucoma. Ophthalmology. 2005;**112**:413-419

[27] Chu TG, Green RL. Suprachoroidal hemorrhage. Survey of Ophthalmology. 1999;**43**:471-486

[28] Wax MB, Kass MA, Kolker AE, Nordlund JR. Anterior lamellar Sclerectomy for Nanophthalmos. Journal of Glaucoma. 1992;**1**:222-227

[29] Brockhurst RJ. Vortex vein decompression for Nanophthalmic uveal effusion. Archives of Ophthalmology. 1980;**98**:1987-1990

[30] Kreiger AE. Wound complications in pars plana vitrectomy. Retinal – Journal of Retinal and Vitreous Disease. 1993;**13**:335-344

[31] Hoffman RS et al. Cataract surgery in the small eye. Journal of Cataract and Refractive Surgery. 2015;**41**:2565-2575

[32] Koc F, Kargi S, Biglan AW, Chu CT, Davis JS. The aetiology in paediatric aphakic glaucoma. Eye. 2006;**20**:1360-1365

[33] Prasad S, Ram J, Sukhija J, Pandav SS, Gupta PC. Cataract surgery in infants with microphthalmos. Graefe's Archive for Clinical and Experimental Ophthalmology. 2015;**253**:739-743

[34] Seki M et al. Nanophthalmos: Quantitative analysis of anterior chamber angle configuration before and after cataract surgery. The British Journal of Ophthalmology. 2012;**96**:1108-1116

[35] Luntz MH, Rosenblatt M. Malignant glaucoma. Survey of Ophthalmology. 1987;**32**:73-93

[36] Yu X et al. Anterior vitrectomy, phacoemulsification cataract extraction and irido-zonulo-hyaloid-vitrectomy in protracted acute angle closure crisis. International Ophthalmology. 2021;**41**:3087-3097

[37] Stürmer J, Kniestedt C, Meier F. Kataraktoperation und kombinierte Katarakt–/Glaukomoperation als augeninnendrucksenkende Maßnahme in Augen mit relativem anterioren Mikrophthalmus. Klinische Monatsblätter für Augenheilkunde. 2005;**222**:206-210

[38] Singh H et al. Refractive outcomes in nanophthalmic eyes after phacoemulsification and implantation of a high-refractive-power foldable intraocular lens. Journal of Cataract and Refractive Surgery. 2015;**41**:2394-2402

[39] Rajendrababu S et al. A comparative study on endothelial cell loss in nanophthalmic eyes undergoing cataract surgery by phacoemulsification. Indian Journal of Ophthalmology. 2021;**69**:279

[40] Wang J, Du E, Tang J. The treatment of malignant glaucoma in nanophthalmos: A case report. BMC Ophthalmology. 2018;**18**:54

[41] Lois N, Wong D, Groenewald C. New surgical approach in the management of pseudophakic malignant glaucoma. Ophthalmology. 2001;**108**:780-783

[42] Kaushik S. Commentary: Malignant glaucoma - have we finally found an answer? Indian Journal of Ophthalmology. 2019;**67**:1206

[43] Żarnowski T et al. Efficacy and safety of a new surgical method to treat malignant glaucoma in pseudophakia. Eye. 2014;**28**:761-764

[44] Long V, Chen S, Hatt SR. Surgical interventions for bilateral congenital cataract. Cochrane Database of Systematic Reviews. 2008;**2008**:D3171

[45] Potop V. Small eye - a small stump which can challenge and tilt a great surgery. Romanian Journal of Ophthalmology. 2016;**60**:138-144

[46] Yu YS, Kim S, Choung HK. Posterior chamber intraocular lens implantation in Pediatric cataract with microcornea and/ or Microphthalmos. Korean Journal of Ophthalmology. 2006;**20**:151

[47] Wendelstein J et al. Project hyperopic power prediction: Accuracy of 13 different concepts for intraocular lens calculation in short eyes. The British Journal of Ophthalmology. 2022;**106**:795-801

[48] Eom Y, Kang S, Song JS, Kim YY, Kim HM. Comparison of Hoffer Q and Haigis formulae for intraocular lens power calculation according to the anterior chamber depth in short eyes. American Journal of Ophthalmology. 2014;**157**:818-824

[49] Moschos M, Chatziralli I, Koutsandrea C. Intraocular lens power calculation in eyes with short axial length. Indian Journal of Ophthalmology. 2014;**62**:692

[50] Voytsekhivskyy OV, Tutchenko L, Hipólito-Fernandes D. Comparison of the Barrett universal II, Kane and VRF-G formulas with existing intraocular lens calculation formulas in eyes with short axial lengths. Eye. 2022;**37**:120-126

[51] Röggla V et al. Accuracy of common IOL power formulas in 611 eyes based on axial length and corneal power ranges. The British Journal of Ophthalmology. 2021;**105**:1661-1665

[52] Hipólito-Fernandes D et al. Anterior chamber depth, lens thickness and

intraocular lens calculation formula accuracy: Nine formulas comparison. The British Journal of Ophthalmology. 2022;**106**:349-355

[53] Yan C, Yao K. Effect of lens vault on the accuracy of intraocular lens calculation formulas in shallow anterior chamber eyes. American Journal of Ophthalmology. 2022;**233**:57-67

[54] Luo Y et al. Comparing the accuracy of new intraocular lens power calculation formulae in short eyes after cataract surgery: A systematic review and meta-analysis. International Ophthalmology. 2022;**42**:1939-1956

[55] Shrivastava A, Nayak S, Mahobia A, Anto M, Pandey P. Accuracy of intraocular lens power calculation formulae in short eyes: A systematic review and meta-analysis. Indian Journal of Ophthalmology. 2022;**70**:740

[56] Lin P et al. A comparative study on the accuracy of IOL calculation formulas in Nanophthalmos and relative anterior Microphthalmos. American Journal of Ophthalmology. 2023;**245**:61-69

[57] Wladis EJ, Gewirtz MB, Guo S. Cataract surgery in the small adult eye. Survey of Ophthalmology. 2006;**51**:153-161

[58] Gayton JL, Sanders VN. Implanting two posterior chamber intraocular lenses in a case of microphthalmos. Journal of Cataract and Refractive Surgery. 1993;**19**:776-777

[59] Mohebbi M et al. Refractive lens exchange and piggyback intraocular lens implantation in nanophthalmos: Visual and structural outcomes. Journal of Cataract and Refractive Surgery. 2017;**43**:1190-1196

Chapter 5

Perspective Chapter: Strategies for Achieving Full-Range of Vision – Multifocal IOLs and Surgical Options for Correcting Residual Refractive Errors

Mateja Jagić, Maja Bohač, Ante Barišić, Dino Šabanović, Sara Blazhevska and Lucija Žerjav

Abstract

Currently, cataract is considered one of the leading causes of visual impairment and blindness globally. Due to the development of surgical techniques and intraocular lenses (IOL) design, patient's demands for complete spectacle independence have grown continuously. Today, the procedure of multifocal IOL implantation is an option for providing a full-range of vision. Although technology has advanced, there are still some drawbacks, such as lower optical quality postoperatively and postoperative residual refractive error, which also greatly reduces spectacle independence, visual quality, and patient satisfaction. Basic options for residual refractive error are the prescription of glasses or contact lenses, but in patients who require life without optical aids, corneal refractive surgery has proven to be a safe and predictable solution. Predominantly, laser-assisted in situ keratomileusis (LASIK) and photorefractive keratectomy (PRK) correction methods are applied, with an emphasis on Aberration-free excimer ablation profiles that do not include wavefront-guided treatments, given the uncertain methods of analyzing higher order aberrations (HOA) in patients with implanted multifocal IOLs.

Keywords: spectacle independence, cataract, multifocal intraocular lenses, residual refractive error, LASIK, PRK

1. Introduction

Cataract is one of the leading causes of blindness globally, with a substantial increase in the prevalence of visual impairment observed in the last three decades. According to the World Health Organization (WHO) report on vision, there are at least 1 billion people with preventable moderate or severe visual impairment or blindness, including 94 million caused by cataract [1, 2]. By 2030, the number of people worldwide aged ≥60 years is estimated to increase 1.4 billion. Given most people over the age of 60 years will develop cataract, the number of people with this condition will also increase substantially [3].

Although many breakthroughs have been made since the inception of Vision 2020 and decreasing blindness prevalence has been achieved during the past decades, the number of blind people continues to increase rapidly [4, 5].

Cataract and presbyopia are the major cause of blindness and vision impairment in the world as a result of the aging population [6]. Along with 94.0 million people visually impaired or blind due to cataract, [2] approximately 1.1. billion people are affected by presbyopia [7]. Currently, around 26% of total population is presbyopic, where the prevalence of presbyopia globally ranges from 43 to 89% for adults aged ≥45 years old [7–13]. About 90% of the global burden of presbyopia occurs in low- and middle-income settings, where presbyopia correction coverage rates are only 10% because of a lack of awareness and access to affordable interventions, and the costs due to uncorrected presbyopia both to the patient and to society are higher than those in high-income settings [13, 14]. Nearly half of the presbyopic patients remain uncorrected, especially in developing countries [9]. As many as 80% of the uncorrected presbyopic patients faced difficulty in performing near-vision-related tasks such as reading, writing, and using mobile devices, which could impact patients' productivity [9, 15]. Likewise, uncorrected presbyopia could pose an economic burden for patients by affecting their work productivity, where they require near vision use to perform work-related tasks. With an increasing population and an aging society, more people will be at risk for common causes of vision loss in the upcoming years [1, 16]; as a prerequisite to combating this growing burden of both cataract and presbyopia, there is a need for greater access to vision care services across the globe for timely screening and optimized correction of aforementioned, especially in the working-age population.

Successful global initiatives targeting improving cataract surgical rate and quality, especially in regions with lower socioeconomic status [17].

The rates of cataract surgery are increasing globally, and postoperative outcomes are improving, yet challenges to reducing the cataract burden remain [18, 19]. Highly cost-effective interventions can offer enormous economic benefits to individuals and nations with relatively low costs. Correcting oncoming presbyopia simultaneously during cataract extraction and intraocular lens (IOL) implantation has been proven to be practical and economical [20–22].

There are various strategies for correcting presbyopia and cataract in clinical practice. Implantation of bilateral monofocal IOL is a conventional surgical strategy for correcting cataract, when targeting emmetropia, it presents lower spectacle independence due to poor intermediate and near visual acuity. Conversely, surgical strategies for both cataract and presbyopia, with higher spectacle independence and greater full-range visual acuity (for distance, intermediate, and near) include, but are not limited to, bilateral implantation of monofocal IOLs targeting monovision, extended depth of focus IOLs, diffractive bifocal IOLs with the same or different near additional power (blended vision), refractive bifocal IOLs, trifocal IOLs [21, 23–25]. Facing diverse strategies, surgeons are expected to customize patient management with satisfactory effectiveness. One of the most common causes of patient dissatisfaction after multifocal intraocular lens (MFIOL) implantation is residual refractive error.

2. Methods

A retrospective study was conducted on patients who underwent implantation of one of the variants of multifocal IOLs during a 10-year period. The visual outcome at distance, intermediate and near, spectacle independence along with patient satisfaction rate and residual refractive error were examined.

Meticulous preoperative examination and careful patient selection with a focus on biometry, ophthalmologic findings, and preoperative astigmatism were performed. The main ophthalmic inclusion criteria were clear cornea without topographic irregularities (irregular or asymmetrical astigmatism), no macular pathology or glaucomatous optic nerve damage, and systemic diseases that might affect postoperative vision (such as diabetes mellitus). Biometry and corneal topography were mandatory and appropriate lens design was chosen according to the amount of corneal astigmatism (toric IOL in astigmatism >0.75D). According to the patient's work habits and demands, one of the listed multifocal IOLs was chosen: diffractive bifocal IOL with low addition (LOW ADD), diffractive extended depth of focus (EDOF), hybrid diffractive EDOF, trifocal, and quadrifocal IOL.

3. Results

3.1 Visual acuity

3.1.1 Distance visual acuity

Our results during a 10-year follow-up showed that all patients had visual acuity better than 0.05 logMar, and almost 70% of patients achieved uncorrected distance visual acuity of 0.00 logMAR, while 10% of patients had uncorrected distance visual acuity worse than 0.1 logMAR. Mean uncorrected distance visual acuity (UDVA) was 0.033 logMar (range 0.03–0.039 between groups) as presented in **Figure 1**, and mean best-corrected distance visual acuity (BCDVA) was 0.024 logMar (range 0.02–0.028 between groups) as presented in **Figure 2**.

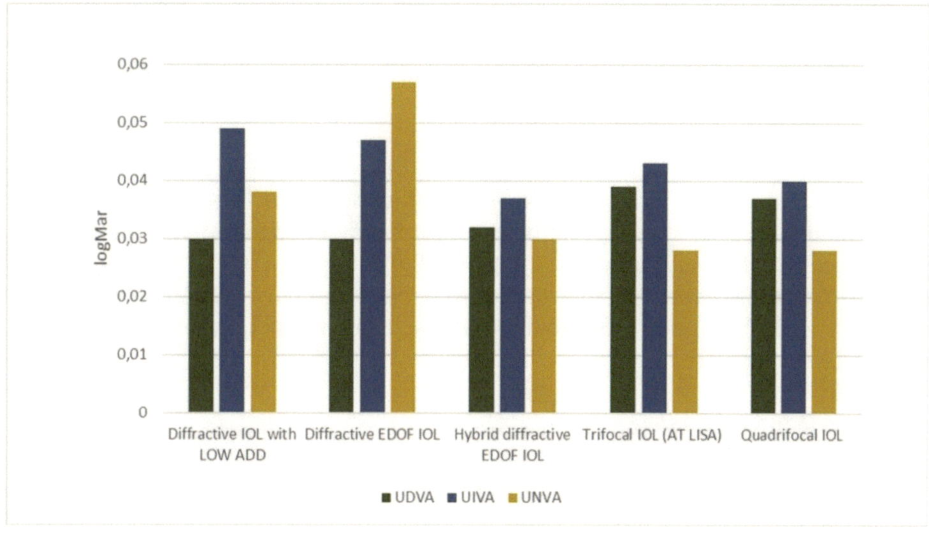

Figure 1.
Comparison of uncorrected visual acuity at distance, intermediate, and near between eyes with different presbyopia-correcting IOLs implanted (values are presented in logMar).

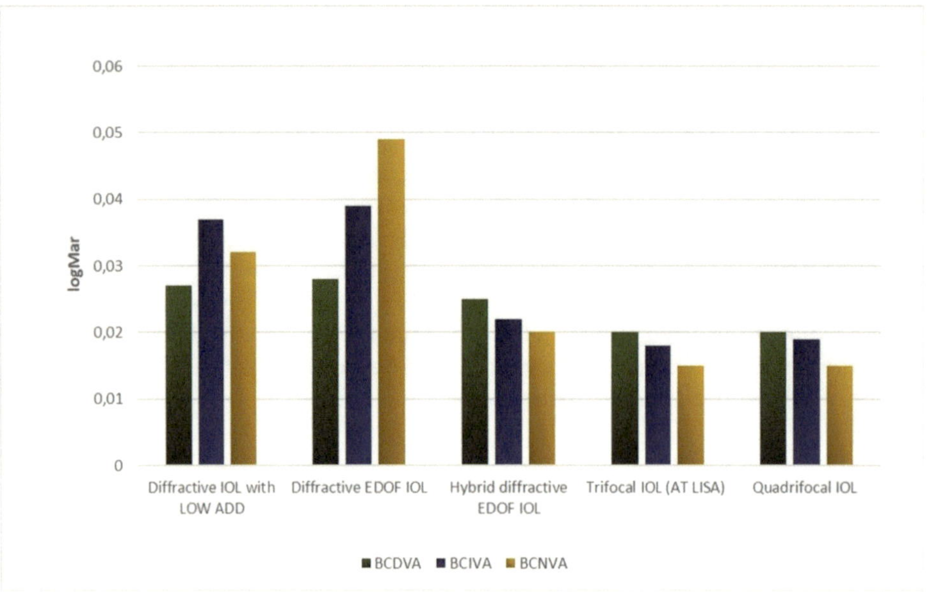

Figure 2.
Comparison of best corrected visual acuity at distance, intermediate, and near between eyes with different presbyopia-correcting IOLs implanted (values are presented in logMar).

3.1.2 Intermediate visual acuity

In the first generations of MFIOLs, the optical design did not allow good vision at intermediate, while, according to our experience, the advancements in technology, mean value of uncorrected visual acuity at intermediate better than 0.1 logMAR was achieved. With newer lens designs such as trifocal, quadrifocal, and EDOF, even better continuity and range of vision at intermediate have been achieved. Mean uncorrected intermediate visual acuity (UIVA) was 0.043 logMar (range 0.037–0.049 between groups), as presented in **Figure 1**, and mean best corrected intermediate visual acuity (BCIVA) was 0.027 logMar (range 0.018–0.038 between groups), as presented in **Figure 2**.

3.1.3 Near visual acuity

Newer generations of lenses have led to an improvement in the quality of vision both near and intermediate, especially for trifocal and quadrifocal IOLs. Mean uncorrected intermediate visual acuity (UNVA) was 0.036 logMar (range 0.028–0.057 between groups), as presented in **Figure 1**, and mean best corrected intermediate visual acuity (BCNVA) was 0.026 logMar (range 0.015–0.049 between groups) as presented in **Figure 2**.

3.2 Spectacle independence

In the literature, there is no clear division between the need for spectacle correction for distance, intermediate, or near. Reported global spectacle independence was ≥80%. In studies where visual acuity for distance, intermediate, and near was separated, spectacle independence was reported for distance in 80% of cases, intermediate in 100% of cases, and near in 70% of cases when implanting various models of IOLs [23, 26–28].

In our previous experience, the need for spectacle correction was highest in patients with refractive bifocal IOLs implanted, in most cases for near-work tasks. After implantation of newer models of presbyopia-correcting IOLs, spectacle independence is significantly greater in comparison to first models of refractive bifocal IOLs, while correction is mostly required for certain activities at intermediate and near distances, depending on IOL design. The highest spectacle independence was observed in patients with hybrid diffractive EDOF, trifocal, and quadrifocal IOLs (**Table 1**).

3.3 Patient satisfaction

Studies have shown that overall patient satisfaction with multifocal lenses is good. Our experiences have shown very high patient satisfaction after implantation of multifocal IOLs (**Figure 3**).

IOL design	Spectacle correction need	
	Overall (%)	For intermediate/near (%)
Diffractive IOL with low add	5.1	2.6
Diffractive EDOF IOL	5.7	2.9
Hybrid diffractive EDOF IOL	2.1	1.2
Trifocal IOL (AT LISA)	2.5	0.8
Quadrifocal IOL	2.6	0.7

Table 1.
Presenting relationship between the need for spectacle correction in total and percentage of spectacle correction need for intermediate and near distance after implantation of various presbyopia-correcting IOLs.

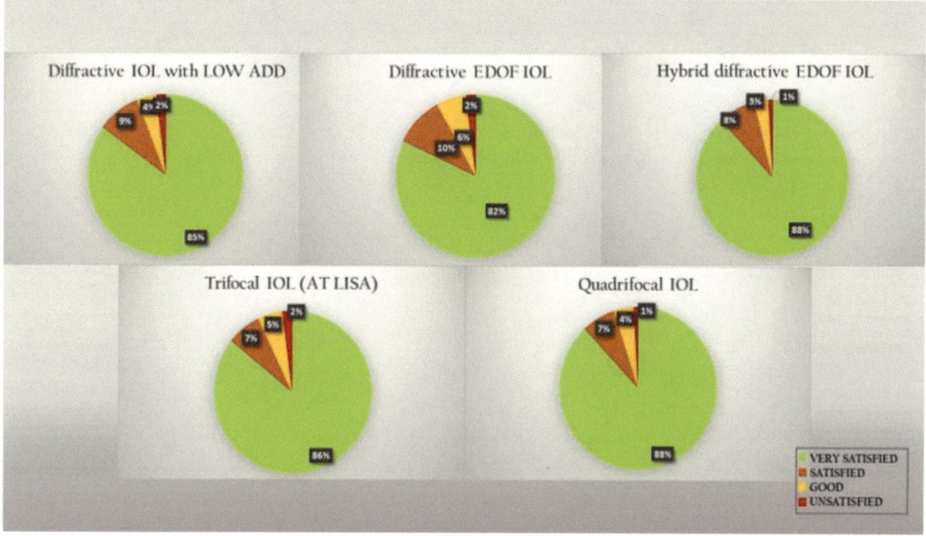

Figure 3.
Graphical presentation of satisfaction rate in patient with different models of presbyopia-correcting IOLs implanted.

Overall patient satisfaction after MFIOL implantation is significantly influenced by preoperative assessment, careful patient selection, and counseling but also varied depending on the preoperative refraction, where the highest satisfaction grade after MFIOL implantation was achieved in patients with high and low hyperopia, as shown in **Table 2**.

The most common causes of patient dissatisfaction after MFIOL implantation are: blurred vision (94.7%) and photic phenomena (38.2%) [29]. The most common causes associated with these symptoms are residual refractive error in 65.5% of eyes, opacification of the posterior capsule in 15.8% of eyes, large pupil diameter in 14.5% of eyes, and wavefront anomalies (HOA) in 11.8% of eyes [30–35]. In our study, visual disturbances were associated with residual refractive error, photic phenomena (halo and glare), and posterior capsule opacifications. Photic phenomena in were also associated with dry eye (5%), and decentration of the IOL (11%). Most common causes of patient dissatisfaction after MFIOL implantation in our facility are shown in **Figure 4**.

Preoperative refraction	Satisfaction grade (scale 1–10)
High hyperopia	9.72 (range 6–10)
Low hyperopia	9.14 (range 4–10)
Plano – presbyopia	8.69 (range 3–10)
High myopia	8.23 (range 4–9)
Low myopia	8.07 (range 2–10)

Table 2.
Grade of patient satisfaction after MFIOL implantation depending on the type of preoperative refractive error.

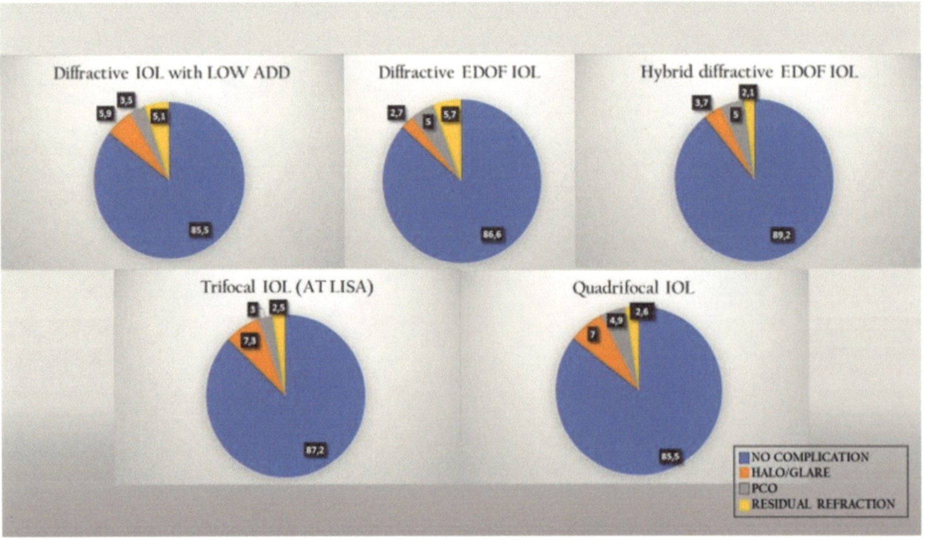

Figure 4.
Graphical presentation of postoperative complication accounted for causes of dissatisfaction in different models of presbyopia-correcting IOLs.

4. Residual refractive error after MFIOL implantation

Despite advances in cataract surgery and intraocular lenses, unsatisfactory postoperative visual outcome may occur as a result of residual refractive error. A recent report analyzed the refractive results of more than 17,000 eyes after cataract surgery and found that emmetropia was achieved in only 55% of eyes. These results emphasized how important residual refractive error is after cataract surgery.

There are various reasons that can lead to residual refractive error after refractive lens replacement. They can be divided into preoperative, intraoperative, and postoperative causes [36].

Preoperative causes include misjudgment of the postoperative effective MFIOL position, errors in measuring the axial length of the eye, inappropriate selection of MFIOL power, limitations of intraocular lens power calculation formulas (especially in extreme ametropia), and lack of precision in MFIOL manufacturing [36, 37]. categories include surgical variation of incision size and position, and capsulorhexis. These factors can affect the final IOL position in the capsular bag and are surgeon-dependent. Unintentional surgically induced astigmatism (SIA) can also be a cause of refractive error after cataract surgery [38].

Postoperative causes that can affect refraction are related to wound healing, changes in corneal curvature, and IOL displacement due to postoperative capsular fibrosis and contraction [38, 39].

Various causes affect not only spherical refractive error but also astigmatism. It is estimated that one-third of patients undergoing cataract surgery or refractive lens exchange (RLE) have corneal astigmatism greater than 1.00D, where the percentage depends on the study population [39, 40]. Although there is an option of toric IOLs for astigmatism correction, despite their noted efficacy, it is reported that up to 47% of eyes had ≥0.5D, and up to 16% of eyes had ≥1.0D of residual astigmatism [41, 42]. Common causes are postoperative IOL rotation, poor IOL position, cumulative errors in power calculating, influence of posterior corneal astigmatism, and pupil size [43].

Literature points out that typical reliability error of subjective refraction ranges from ±0.34D to ±0.51D [44, 45], and it is affected by various factors such as attention, duration of a concentrated visual task (e.g., close work, pressure on eyelids, and pupil size/depth of field) [46–48]. Small shifts in the sphere, amount of astigmatism, and its axis can be related to these factors. Postoperative refractive error ≥ 0.50D is considered clinically significant, where causes of unexpected spherical errors are easily identified; however, the same cannot apply to unexpected astigmatic errors postoperatively [49].

After implantation of spherical MFIOLs, the axis of SIA did not correlate with the axis or amount of preoperative astigmatism. However, the severity of SIA was related to the axis of preoperative astigmatism. When preoperative astigmatism is low (≤1.00D), and predominantly against the rule (ATR), SIA can be up to 1.00D [50].

4.1 Keratorefractive surgical strategy for correcting residual refractive error after MFIOL implantation

Correction of residual refractive errors after MFIOL implantation initially includes prescription of glasses or contact lenses. In the case of the patient's desire for complete spectacle/contact lens independence, either corneal surgery (incisional procedures, excimer laser correction procedures) or intraocular surgery (IOL exchange, piggyback IOL implantation) is considered. In the case of low residual astigmatic error, the option of incisional techniques (LRI, AK) can be considered, while in the case of high ametropia or unavailability of technology, new intraocular procedures are recommended. Excimer laser correction of residual refractive errors in pseudophakic patients proved to be safe and predictable as an adjustment of final results. The advantages compared to intraocular surgery are greater flexibility achievement of satisfactory results, and the avoidance of trauma caused by additional intraocular procedures.

The safety of LASIK and PRK in pseudophakic patients has already been reported in several studies. In general, the procedure is recommended to be performed at least 6–12 weeks after intraocular procedure due to potential complications related to corneal incision integrity, subclinical corneal edema, and IOL stability. If a residual refractive error is expected during the preoperative examination, a corneal flap can be made before the lens is implanted (a procedure called Bioptics). This enables earlier and less traumatic correction of residual ametropia after stabilizing the refractive error. Before planning excimer laser correction, there are challenges in assessing residual refractive error due to the existence of multiple focal points (causing artifacts in subjective refraction) and changes in refraction depending on lighting conditions and pupil size.

According to the published literature, automatic refractometry, which is often used as a starting point in determining subjective refraction, shows a tendency for more negative values (~ 1.0D for sphere; ~ 0.5D for cylinder), as well as retinoscopy (≤ 0.5D for sphere and cylinder). Different methods have been proposed for the accurate assessment of subjective refraction in patients after MFIOL implantation. Currently, there is a consensus that keratometric values are the starting point in refraction assessment, given that IOL implantation does not have a significant impact on them, and then visual acuity must be checked by evaluating the defocusing curve (**Figure 5**).

Currently, most authors suggest aspheric treatments for the correction of residual refractive errors after MFIOL implantation, since Hartmann-Shack aberrometers are not able to analyze the exact values of the higher order aberrations (HOA) and

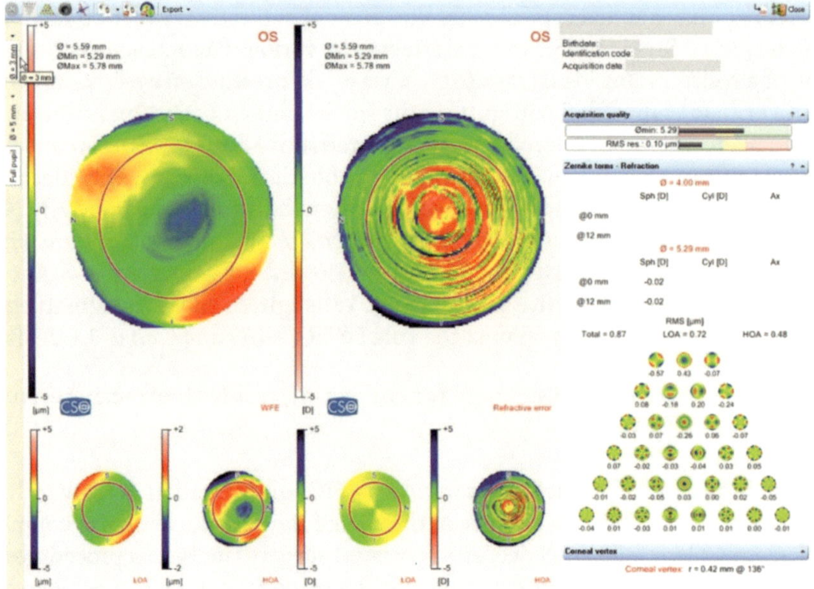

Figure 5.
Aberrometry report in patient with implanted MFIOL.

scattering due to the limitation imposed by the lens sampling. Pyramidal aberrometers, such as Schwind Peramis (Schwind Eye Tech Solutions, Kleinostheim, Germany), in contrast to other methods, is sampling wavefront in the very last stage of the optical path, and is sampled with 45,000 points at maximum pupil dilation, which corresponds to a much higher resolution. Therefore, it could provide better HOA analysis after MFIOL implantation [51–55].

According to our experience, the percentage of patients who required additional correction postoperatively in most cases correlated with the percentage of patients who opted for excimer laser enhancement after MFIOL implantation, with variations between different types of IOLs. Lower percentage of LASIK enhancements in diffractive LOW ADD and EDOF group was due to the fact that overall spectacle correction was required mostly for intermediate and/or near-work tasks, which was proactively discussed with patients before deciding on lens design. Higher percentage of surgical enhancement observed in patients with implanted trifocal and quadrifocal IOLs has been reported due to higher patient demands for better vision, regardless of working distance (**Figure 6**).

At our center, 42 patients (eyes) out of 2119 MFIOL-implanted eyes opted for LASIK enhancement with the Free Aberration™ program (Schwind AMARIS 750S and 1050RS; Schwind Eye Tech Solutions, Kleinostheim, Germany) 6 months after MFIOL implantation (**Table 3**).

The mean spherical and cylindrical correction values were + 0.45D (range – 1.75D to +2.00D) and – 0.91D (range – 3.00D to 0D), and after LASIK they decreased to +0.05D (range from −0.25D to +1.00D) and – 0.18D (range from −0.50D to 0 D) (**Figure 7**). Corrections were based on the best subjective refraction.

Figure 8 shows that there was a simultaneous improvement in visual acuity with a reduction in residual refractive error for all distances.

See **Figure 9**.

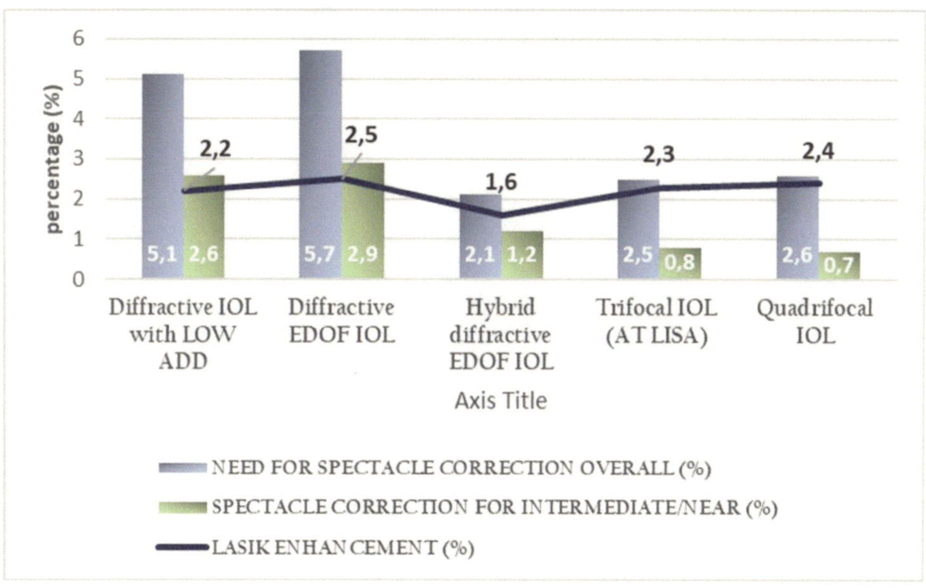

Figure 6.
Graphical presentation of spectacle correction and excimer laser enhancement rate in groups with different presbyopia-correcting IOLs implanted.

IOL design	N (Eyes) implanted/ N (Eyes) treated w. Lasik	%
Diffractive IOL with low add	588/13	2.21
Diffractive EDOF IOL	252/6	2.50
Hybrid diffractive EDOF IOL	984/16	1.62
Trifocal IOL (AT LISA)	211/5	2.36
Quadrifocal IOL	84/2	2.38

Table 3.
Number and percentage of eyes treated with LASIK after implantation of different presbyopia-correcting IOLs.

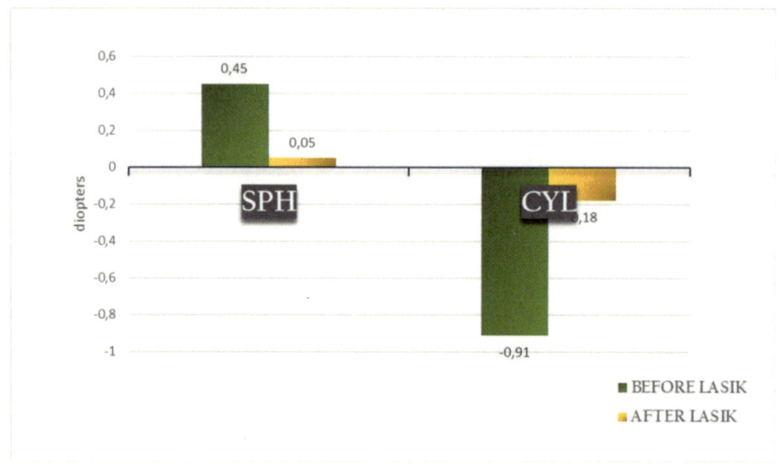

Figure 7.
Comparison of sphere and cylinder correction before and after LASIK enhancement.

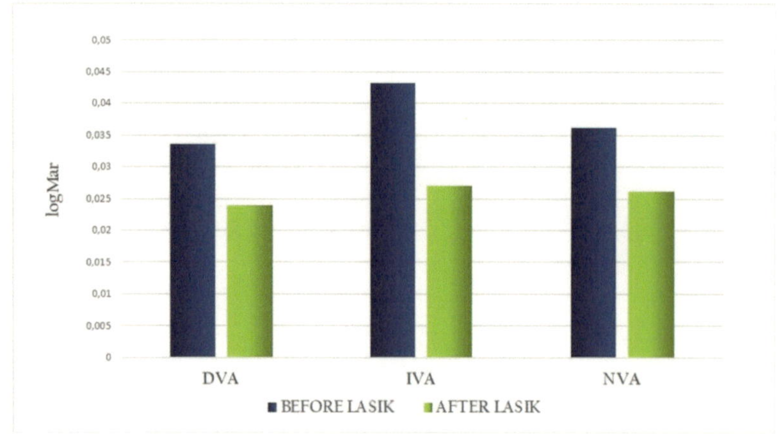

Figure 8.
Uncorrected visual acuity on distance, intermediate, and near before and after LASIK enhancement.

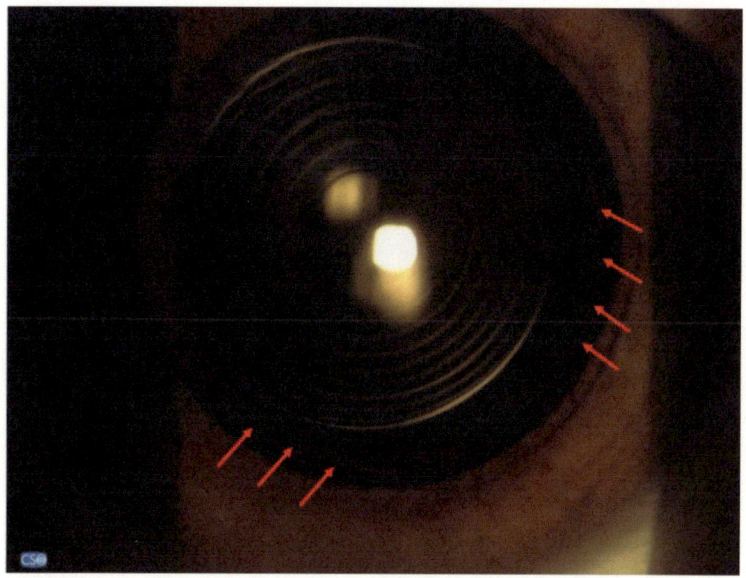

Figure 9.
Slit lamp presentation of well-positioned corneal flap (red arrows) 1 month postoperatively in patient with a previously implanted MFIOL.

5. Conclusion

Modern cataract surgery with implantation of multifocal intraocular lenses continuously raises patients' expectations to complete spectacle independence. Advances in technology have enabled cataract surgery to develop from being concerned primarily with correcting aphakia into a procedure refined to achieve the best possible postoperative refractive result. Today, after MFIOL implantation, patients have satisfactory visual acuity at all working distances and a high percentage of independence from glasses, and overall patient satisfaction is high.

Despite surgical technique and IOL technology development, refractive surprise occurs occasionally causing patient's dissatisfaction after MFIOL implantation. Therefore, enhancements are often necessary to provide spectacle independence for distance and near vision for patients after MFIOL implantation. In addition to conservative treatments (correction with glasses and contact lenses), residual refractive error can be safely and predictably treated with excimer laser correction surgery, where LASIK and PRK are the most commonly used methods in clinical practice. The advantages compared to other surgical options are greater flexibility, achieving good and predictable results and avoidance of trauma caused by additional intraocular procedures.

Further improvements in MFIOL technology, biometric technology and IOL formulas, preoperative counseling, postoperative assessment, and management of residual refractive error are needed to further improve outcome and increase patient satisfaction.

Author details

Mateja Jagić*, Maja Bohač, Ante Barišić, Dino Šabanović, Sara Blazhevska and Lucija Žerjav
University Eye Hospital Svjetlost, Zagreb, Croatia

*Address all correspondence to: mateja.jagic@svjetlost.hr

References

[1] WHO: World Report on Vision. Magnitude, temporal trends, and projections of the global prevalence of blindness and distance and near vision impairment: A systematic review and meta-analysis; 2019

[2] Steinmetz JD, Bourne RRA, Briant PS, et al. Causes of blindness and vision impairment in 2020 and trends over 30 years, and prevalence of avoidable blindness in relation to VISION 2020: The right to sight: An analysis for the global burden of disease study. The Lancet Global Health. 2021;**9**:e144-e160

[3] World Health Organization. Decade of Healthy Ageing: Baseline Report. Geneva: World Health Organization; 2020. Licence: CC BY-NC-SA 3.0 IGO

[4] Flaxman SR, Bourne RRA, Resnikoff S, Ackland P, Braithwaite T, Cicinelli MV, et al. Global causes of blindness and distance vision impairment 1990-2020: A systematic review and meta-analysis. The Lancet Global Health. 2017;**5**:e1221-e1234

[5] Taylor HR. Global blindness: The Progress we are making and still need to make. Asia-Pacific Journal of Ophthalmology. 2019;**8**:424-428

[6] Bourne R, Steinmetz JD, Flaxman S, et al. Trends in prevalence of blindness and distance and near vision impairment over 30 years: An analysis for the global burden of disease study. The Lancet Global Health. 2021;**9**:e130-e143. DOI: 10.1016/s2214-109x(20)30425-3

[7] Bourne RRA, Flaxman SR, Braithwaite T, et al. Magnitude, temporal trends, and projections of the global prevalence of blindness and distance and near vision impairment: A systematic review and meta-analysis. The Lancet Global Health. 2017;**5**(9):e888-e897. DOI: 10.1016/S2214-109X(17)30293-0

[8] Hookway LA, Frazier M, Rivera N, Ramson P, Carballo L, Naidoo K. Population-based study of presbyopia in Nicaragua. Clinical & Experimental Optometry. 2016;**99**(6):559-563. DOI: 10.1111/cxo.12402

[9] Holden BA, Fricke TR, Ho SM, et al. Global vision impairment due to uncorrected presbyopia. Archives of Ophthalmology. 2008;**126**(12):1731-1739. DOI: 10.1001/archopht.126.12.1731

[10] Mitchell JP, Williams N, Martin R, et al. The Venezuela eye evaluation study. Journal of the National Medical Association. 2008;**100**(4):435-438. DOI: 10.1016/S0027-9684(15)31278-5

[11] Cunha CC, Berezovsky A, Furtado JM, et al. Presbyopia and ocular conditions causing near vision impairment in older adults from the Brazilian Amazon region. American Journal of Ophthalmology. 2018;**196**:72-81. DOI: 10.1016/j.ajo.2018.08.012

[12] Census US. U.S.: Estimated 2010 Prevalence of Presbyopia in Adults Aged 45 or Older; census Figure Applied to Prevalence Number to Calculate Rate Bonilla-Warford N; "What to Do with 'New' Presbyopes." Review of Optometry. 2010:42

[13] Fricke TR, Tahhan N, Resnikoff S, et al. Global prevalence of presbyopia and vision impairment from uncorrected presbyopia: Systematic review, meta-analysis, and modelling. Ophthalmology. 2018;**125**:1492-1499

[14] Donaldson KEJ. The economic impact of presbyopia. Journal of Refractive Surgery. 2021;**37**:S17-S19

[15] Berdahl J, Bala C, Dhariwal M, Lemp-Hull J, Thakker D, Jawla S. Patient and economic burden of presbyopia: A systematic literature review. Clinical Ophthalmology. 2020 Oct;**22**(14):3439-3450. DOI: 10.2147/OPTH.S269597

[16] Bourne RRA, Flaxman SR, Braithwaite T, Cicinelli MV, Das A, Jonas JB, et al. Magnitude, temporal trends, and projections of the global prevalence of blindness and distance and near vision impairment: A systematic review and meta-analysis. The Lancet Global Health. 2017;**5**:e888-e897

[17] Ramke J, Silva JC, Gichangi M, Ravilla T, Burn H, Buchan JC, et al. Cataract services for all: Strategies for equitable access from a global modified Delphi process. PLOS Global Public Health. 2023;**3**(2):e0000631. DOI: 10.1371/journal.pgph.0000631

[18] Lee CM, Afshari NA. The global state of cataract blindness. Current Opinion in Ophthalmology. 2017;**28**:98-103

[19] Ramke J, Evans JR, Gilbert CE. Reducing inequity of cataract blindness and vision impairment is a global priority, but where is the evidence? British Journal of Ophthalmology. 2018;**102**(9):1179-1181. DOI: 10.1136/bjophthalmol-2018-311985

[20] Kim TI, Alió Del Barrio JL, Wilkins M, Cochener B, Ang M. Refractive surgery. Lancet. 2019;**393**(10185):2085-2098. DOI: 10.1016/S0140-6736(18)33209-4

[21] Wolffsohn JS, Davies LN. Presbyopia: Effectiveness of correction strategies. Progress in Retinal and Eye Research. 2019;**68**:124-143. DOI: 10.1016/j.preteyeres.2018.09.004. Epub 2018 Sep 19

[22] Kollbaum PS, Bradley A. Correction of presbyopia: Old problems with old (and new) solutions. Clinical & Experimental Optometry. 2020;**103**(1):21-30. DOI: 10.1111/cxo.12987. Epub 2019 Nov 17

[23] de Silva SR, Evans JR, Kirthi V, Ziaei M, Leyland M. Multifocal versus monofocal intraocular lenses after cataract extraction. Cochrane Database of Systematic Reviews. 2016;**12**(12):CD003169. DOI: 10.1002/14651858.CD003169.pub4

[24] Hu JQ, Sarkar R, Sella R, Murphy JD, Afshari NA. Cost-effectiveness analysis of multifocal intraocular lenses compared to Monofocal intraocular lenses in cataract surgery. American Journal of Ophthalmology. 2019;**208**:305-312. DOI: 10.1016/j.ajo.2019.03.019. Epub 2019 Mar 21

[25] Rampat R, Gatinel D. Multifocal and extended depth-of-focus intraocular lenses in 2020. Ophthalmology. 2021;**128**(11):e164-e185. DOI: 10.1016/j.ophtha.2020.09.026. Epub 2020 Sep 25

[26] Alio JL, Plaza-Puche AB, Férnandez-Buenaga R, Pikkel J, Maldonado M. Multifocal intraocular lenses: An overview. Survey of Ophthalmology. 2017;**62**(5):611-634. DOI: 10.1016/j.survophthal.2017.03.005. Epub 2017 Mar 31

[27] Khandelwal SS, Jun JJ, Mak S, Booth MS, Shekelle PG. Effectiveness of multifocal and monofocal intraocular lenses for cataract surgery and lens replacement: A systematic review and meta-analysis. Graefe's Archive for Clinical and Experimental Ophthalmology. 2019;**257**(5):863-875. DOI: 10.1007/s00417-018-04218-6. Epub 2019 Jan 10

[28] Kelava L, Barić H, Bušić M, Čima I, Trkulja V. Monovision versus multifocality for presbyopia: Systematic

review and meta-analysis of randomized controlled trials. Advances in Therapy. 2017;**34**(8):1815-1839. DOI: 10.1007/s12325-017-0579-7. Epub 2017 Jul 3

[29] de Vries NE, Webers CA, Touwslager WR, Bauer NJ, de Brabander J, Berendschot TT, et al. Dissatisfaction after implantation of multifocal intraocular lenses. Journal of Cataract and Refractive Surgery. 2011;**37**(5):859-865. DOI: 10.1016/j.jcrs.2010.11.032. Epub 2011 Mar 11

[30] Ortiz D, Alió JL, Bernabéu G, Pongo V. Optical performance of monofocal and multifocal intraocular lenses in the human eye. Journal of Cataract and Refractive Surgery. 2008;**34**(5):755-762. DOI: 10.1016/j.jcrs.2007.12.038

[31] Montés-Micó R, España E, Bueno I, Charman WN, Menezo JL. Visual performance with multifocal intraocular lenses: Mesopic contrast sensitivity under distance and near conditions. Ophthalmology. 2004;**111**(1):85-96. DOI: 10.1016/S0161-6420(03)00862-5

[32] Pieh S, Lackner B, Hanselmayer G, Zöhrer R, Sticker M, Weghaupt H, et al. Halo size under distance and near conditions in refractive multifocal intraocular lenses. The British Journal of Ophthalmology. 2001;**85**(7):816-821. DOI: 10.1136/bjo.85.7.816

[33] Osher RH. Negative dysphotopsia: Long-term study and possible explanation for transient symptoms. Journal of Cataract and Refractive Surgery. 2008;**34**(10):1699-1707. DOI: 10.1016/j.jcrs.2008.06.026

[34] Elgohary MA, Beckingsale AB. Effect of posterior capsular opacification on visual function in patients with monofocal and multifocal intraocular lenses. Eye (London, England). 2008;**22**(5):613-619. DOI: 10.1038/sj.eye.6702661. Epub 2006 Dec 22

[35] Lee ES, Lee SY, Jeong SY, Moon YS, Chin HS, Cho SJ, et al. Effect of postoperative refractive error on visual acuity and patient satisfaction after implantation of the Array multifocal intraocular lens. Journal of Cataract and Refractive Surgery. 2005;**31**(10):1960-1965. DOI: 10.1016/j.jcrs.2005.03.062

[36] Norrby S. Sources of error in intraocular lens power calculation. Journal of Cataract and Refractive Surgery. 2008;**34**(3):368-376. DOI: 10.1016/j.jcrs.2007.10.031

[37] Alio JL, Abdelghany AA, Fernández-Buenaga R. Management of residual refractive error after cataract surgery. Current Opinion in Ophthalmology. 2014;**25**(4):291-297. DOI: 10.1097/ICU.0000000000000067

[38] Kawahara A, Kurosaka D, Yoshida A. Comparison of surgically induced astigmatism between one-handed and two-handed cataract surgery techniques. Clinical Ophthalmology. 2013;**7**:1967-1972. DOI: 10.2147/opth.s52415. Epub 2013 Oct 2

[39] Ferrer-Blasco T, Montés-Micó R, Peixoto-de-Matos SC, González-Méijome JM, Cerviño A. Prevalence of corneal astigmatism before cataract surgery. Journal of Cataract and Refractive Surgery. 2009;**35**(1):70-75. DOI: 10.1016/j.jcrs.2008.09.027

[40] Michelitsch M, Ardjomand N, Vidic B, Wedrich A, Steinwender G. Prävalenz und Altersabhängigkeit von kornealem Astigmatismus bei Patienten vor Kataraktchirurgie [prevalence and age-related changes of corneal astigmatism in patients before cataract surgery]. Der Ophthalmologe.

2017;**114**(3):247-251. German. DOI: 10.1007/s00347-016-0323-8

[41] Visser N, Bauer NJC, Nuijts RMMA. Toric intraocular lenses: Historical overview, patient selection, IOL calculation, surgical techniques, clinical outcomes, and complications. Journal of Cataract and Refractive Surgery. 2013;**39**:624-637

[42] Waltz KL, Featherstone K, Tsai L, Trentacost D. Clinical outcomes of TECNIS toric intraocular lens implantation after cataract removal in patients with corneal astigmatism. Ophthalmology. 2015;**122**:39-47

[43] Garzón N, Rodríguez-Vallejo M, Carmona D, Calvo-Sanz JA, Poyales F, Palomino C, et al. Comparing surgically induced astigmatism calculated by means of simulated keratometry versus total corneal refractive power. European Journal of Ophthalmology. 2018;**28**(5):573-581. DOI: 10.1177/1120672118757666. Epub 2018 Mar 22

[44] Jennings JAM, Charman WN. A comparison of errors in some methods of subjective refraction. Ophthalmic Optician. 1973;**13**:11-18

[45] Leinonen LE, Laatikainen L. Repeatability (test-retest variability) of refractive error measurement in clinical settings. Acta Ophthalmologica. 2006;**84**:532-536. DOI: 10.1111/j.1600-0420.2006.00695.x

[46] Ford JG, Davis RM, Reed JW, et al. Bilateral monocular diplopia associated with lid positionduring near work. Cornea. 1997;**16**:525-530

[47] Golnik KC, Eggenberger E. Symptomatic corneal topographic change induced by reading in downgaze. Journal of Neuro-Ophthalmology. 2001;**21**:199-204

[48] Grey C, Yap M. Influence of lid position on astigmatism. American Journal of Optometry and Physiological Optics. 1986;**63**:966-969

[49] Abdelghany AA, Alio JL. Surgical options for correction of refractive error following cataract surgery. Eye and Vision (London). 2014;**1**:2. DOI: 10.1186/s40662-014-0002-2

[50] Theodoulidou S, Asproudis I, Athanasiadis A, Kokkinos M, Aspiotis M. Comparison of surgically induced astigmatism among different surgeons performing the same incision. International Journal of Ophthalmology. 2017;**10**(6):1004-1007. DOI: 10.18240/ijo.2017.06.26

[51] Bohač M, Barišić A, Patel S, Gabrić N. Multifocal intraocular lenses: Postimplantation residual refractive error. Multifocal intraocular lenses. In: Alió JL, Pikkel J. ur, editors. Multifocal Lenses: The Art and the Practice. Cham: Springer International Publishing; 2019. pp. 93-101

[52] Cade F, Cruzat A, Paschalis EI, Espírito Santo L, Pineda R. Analysis of four aberrometers for evaluating lower and higher order aberrations. PLoS One. 2013;**8**(1):e54990. DOI: 10.1371/journal.pone.0054990. Epub 2013 Jan 22

[53] Plaza-Puche AB, Salerno LC, Versaci F, Romero D, Alio JL. Clinical evaluation of the repeatability of ocular aberrometry obtained with a new pyramid wavefront sensor. European Journal of Ophthalmology. 2019;**29**(6):585-592. DOI: 10.1177/1120672118816060. Epub 2018 Dec 5

[54] Maurino V, Allan BD, Rubin GS, Bunce C, Xing W, Findl O, et al. Quality

of vision after bilateral multifocal intraocular lens implantation: A randomized trial—AT LISA 809M versus AcrySof ReSTOR SN6AD1. Ophthalmology. 2015;**122**(4):700-710

[55] Muftuoglu O, Prasher P, Chu C, et al. Laser in situ keratomileusis for residual refractive errors after apodized diffractive multifocal intraocular lens implantation. Journal of Cataract & Refractive Surgery. 2009;**35**(6):1063-1071